28ª

99QP

CLINICAL PROGRESS IN
CARDIOVASCULAR DISEASE

CONTRIBUTORS

EDGAR V. ALLEN, M.D., Division of Medicine, Mayo Clinic, Rochester, Minn.

MARK D. ALTSCHULE, M.D., Assistant Professor of Medicine, Harvard Medical School, and Visiting Physician and Research Associate, Beth Israel Hospital, Boston; Director of Internal Medicine and Research in Clinical Physiology, McLean Hospital, Waverly, Mass.

EDWARD F. BLAND, M.D., Physician, Massachusetts General Hospital; Visiting Physician, House of the Good Samaritan; Clinical Associate in Medicine, Harvard Medical School, Boston, Mass.

CLARENCE E. DE LA CHAPELLE, M.D., Professor of Medicine and Associate Dean, New York University Post-Graduate Medical School; Visiting Physician, Fourth (New York University) Medical Division, Bellevue Hospital; Director of Medicine, Lenox Hill Hospital, New York, N. Y.

DAVID COLMAN, B.S., The Donner Laboratory of Medical Physics and the Radiation Laboratory, University of California, Berkeley, Calif.

A. CARLTON ERNSTENE, M.D., Chief of Staff, Division of Medicine, Cleveland Clinic, Cleveland, Ohio.

JOHN W. GOFMAN, M.D., PH.D., Assistant Professor of Medical Physics, Division of Medical Physics, University of California, Berkeley; Clinical Instructor in Medicine, University of California Medical School, San Francisco, Calif.

VIRGIL HERRING, M.S., The Donner Laboratory of Medical Physics and the Radiation Laboratory, University of California, Berkeley, Calif.

HARDIN B. JONES, PH.D., Associate Professor of Medical Physics and Physiology, University of California, Berkeley, Calif.

LOUIS N. KATZ, M.D., Cardiovascular Department, Medical Research Institute, Michael Reese Hospital, Chicago, Ill.

ANCEL KEYS, PH.D., LABORATORY OF PHYSIOLOGICAL HYGIENE, University of Minnesota, Minneapolis, Minn.

FRANK, LINDGREN, B.S., Research Assistant in Medical Physics, Division of Medical Physics, University of California, Berkeley, Calif.

THOMAS, P. LYON, M.D., Research Associate in Medical Physics, The Radiation Laboratory, University of California, Berkeley; Clinical Instructor in Medicine, University of California Medical School, San Francisco, Calif.

O. ALAN ROSE, M.D., Assistant Professor of Clinical Medicine, New York University College of Medicine; Assistant Visiting Physician, Third (New York University) Medical Division, Bellevue Hospital and University Hospital, New York, N. Y.

BEVERLY STRISOWER, B.S., Research Assistant in Medical Physics, Division of Medical Physics, University of California, Berkeley, Calif.

CLINICAL PROGRESS IN CARDIOVASCULAR DISEASE

Edited by HERRMAN L. BLUMGART, M.D.

*Physician-in-Chief, Beth Israel Hospital, and Professor
of Medicine, Harvard Medical School, Boston, Mass.*

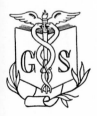

GRUNE & STRATTON · New York

1952

Contents

INTRODUCTION, *Herrman L. Blumgart* 1

ATHEROSCLEROSIS. A SYMPOSIUM 5

   INTRODUCTION, *Edgar V. Allen* 5

   EXPERIMENTAL ATHEROSCLEROSIS, *Louis N. Katz* 9

   HUMAN ATHEROSCLEROSIS AND THE DIET, *Ancel Keys* 33

   BLOOD LIPIDS AND HUMAN ATHEROSCLEROSIS, *John W. Gofman, Hardin B. Jones, Thomas P. Lyon, Frank Lindgren, Beverly Strisower, David Colman and Virgil Herring* 39

   THE MANAGEMENT OF ACUTE CARDIAC EMERGENCIES, *Clarence E. de la Chapelle and O. Alan Rose* 67

   SURGERY FOR MITRAL STENOSIS. A REVIEW OF PROGRESS, *Edward F. Bland* 87

   THE MANAGEMENT OF CARDIAC PATIENTS IN RELATION TO SURGERY, *A. Carlton Ernstene* 106

   EMOTION AND THE CIRCULATION, *Mark D. Altschule* 118

INDEX 137

Introduction

PROGRESS in our knowledge of the heart and blood vessels has been gratifying. But as our perception of the interplay between the circulation and the functions of every organ has widened, cardiovascular disease has almost ceased to be a specialty; rather, it embraces and is embraced by all of medicine. Our comprehension of the physiology and disorders of the cardiovascular system has drawn on all medical disciplines and fields of biology and science. Advances in metabolism, nutrition, electrophysics, radioisotopes, blood coagulation, bacteriology, immunology, genetics, physical and biochemistry are but a few disciplines that may be cited. For an investigator to be conversant with the main trends of studies even in neighboring fields is not only frequently difficult but, indeed, impracticable. Moreover, the clinician is confronted by the even more difficult decision as to whether knowledge has reached the stage where it may justifiably and safely be applied to the improvement of diagnosis and treatment of his patient.

Those responsible for the editorial policy of CIRCULATION wisely discerned that many important purposes could be served by authoritative critical reviews of our accumulated knowledge. In this way the efforts of investigators would be facilitated by summaries of specialized knowledge appearing in fragments in many different journals by numerous workers. Investigation in basic sciences would be aided by clinical surveys and, conversely, the clinician would profit by authoritative discussions of the basic knowledge which is fundamental to the understanding of clinical phenomena. Thus, a new section, "Clinical Progress," was inaugurated in December 1950 as a monthly feature of CIRCULATION, and it is from these sections that this volume is drawn.

In cardiology, as in medicine in general, many issues remain sub-judice. Critical appraisal of the current status of such problems promotes progress. By clearly defining the gaps in our knowledge, further

1

speculation, clinical observation, and productive research are stimulated.

It is hardly surprising, when one considers the above manifold functions of "Clinical Progress," that a wide diversity of contributions has appeared. With the appearance of the present volume, the following have been published:

The Modern Treatment of Coronary Thrombosis with Myocardial Infarction, *Irving S. Wright* (December 1950)

The Patent Ductus Arteriosus. Observations from 412 Surgically Treated Cases, *Robert E. Gross and Luther A. Longino* (January 1951)

Renal Factor in Congestive Heart Failure, *Eugene A. Stead, Jr.* (February 1951)

Emotion and the Circulation, *Mark D. Altschule* (March 1951)

Angiography, *Charles T. Dotter, Israel Steinberg and Robert B. Ball* (April 1951)

The Effects of Cortisone and ACTH on the Acute Phase of Rheumatic Fever, *Arlie R. Barnes* (May 1951)

Clinical Aspects of Mercurial Diuretics, *C. Thorpe Ray and George E. Burch* (June 1951)

Angiocardiography, *Charles T. Dotter and Israel Steinberg* (July 1951)

Chronic Constrictive Pericarditis, *Paul D. White* (August 1951)

The Management of Cardiac Patients in Relation to Surgery, *A. Carlton Ernstene* (September 1951)

Anticoagulant Therapy in Peripheral Vascular Disease, *Nelson W. Barker* (October 1951)

The Management of Acute Cardiac Emergencies, *Clarence E. de la Chapelle and O. Alan Rose* (November 1951)

Cardiac Asthma, *Thomas A. Lombardo and Tinsley R. Harrison* (December 1951)

Atherosclerosis. A Symposium, *Edgar V. Allen, Guest Editor, and Louis N. Katz, Ancel Keys and John W. Gofman et al., participants* (January 1952)

Surgery for Mitral Stenosis. A Review of Progress, *Edward F. Bland* (February 1952)

Needless Restrictions Imposed on Cardiac Patients, *Robert L. Levy* (March 1952)

The Functional Importance of Coronary Collaterals, *Carl J. Wiggers* (April 1952)

The Specific Treatment of Syphilitic Aortitis, *R. H. Kampmeier and Hugh J. Morgan* (May 1952)

The Anesthetic Management of Patients with Heart Disease, *Robert D. Dripps and Leroy D. Vandam* (June 1952)

Sympathectomy for Essential Hypertension, *Edgar V. Allen* (July 1952)

The essays of the present volume were chosen because they are pertinent to significant problems of current interest and because of their practical usefulness. The first, on atherosclerosis, deals with a subject which is being investigated vigorously with diverse technics and which is inevitably controversial at the present stage of its development. The authoritative opinions of investigators approaching the problem from different angles under the editorial leadership of Dr. Edgar V. Allen has evoked much discussion. Similarly, "Surgery for Mitral Stenosis. A Review of Progress," by Dr. Edward F. Bland, with his conservative, encouraging evaluation of the clinical benefits, has been informative to all interested in this field. The essays by Drs. Clarence E. de la Chapelle and O. Alan Rose, by Dr. A. Carlton Ernstene and Dr. Mark D. Altschule bring up to date the accumulated knowledge in areas which are part of the armamentarium of every clinician.

HERRMAN L. BLUMGART, M.D.

Boston, March 1952

Atherosclerosis. A Symposium

Guest Editor: Edgar V. Allen, M.D.
Participants: Louis N. Katz, M.D., Ancel Keys, Ph.D., and John W. Gofman, M.D., Ph.D.

Introduction

By Edgar V. Allen, M.D.

This symposium is the result of participation by Doctors Katz, Keys, and Gofman in a discussion of various aspects of atherosclerosis which was a part of a postgraduate course in Peripheral Vascular Diseases, conducted under the auspices of the American College of Physicians, by the Staff of the Mayo Clinic, the Faculty of the University of Minnesota (Mayo Foundation for Medical Education and Research), and invited speakers, at Rochester, Minnesota, in the fall of 1950.

The material presented at that time was so important and so timely that failure to record it in the medical literature would be, obviously, an error of great magnitude. With the consent of Dr. Herrman L. Blumgart, I asked that these manuscripts be prepared for publication in Circulation. I need not emphasize here the importance of atherosclerosis, except to say that it is the most important disease in America and in areas where economics, diet and ways of life are similar to ours. It is my belief that this symposium constitutes the most important published work on atherosclerosis in medical history. For the clinicians, who must interpret advances in the laboratories for the benefit of their patients, I have requested that Doctor Katz, Doctor Keys and Doctor Gofman answer three specific questions:

Questions

1. *Has It Been Proved That Human Atherosclerosis Results from the Ingestion of Cholesterol and/or Fat?*

5

2. *In the Light of Present Knowledge, Is It Probable That Human Atherosclerosis Is Caused by the Ingestion of Cholesterol and/or Fat?*

3. *Would You Recommend That a Patient Who Has Clinical Evidence of Atherosclerosis Have His Diet Sharply Restricted in Cholesterol and Fat?*

Answers

Louis N. Katz, M.D.

1. I would say the answer is yes. This is not to be taken, however, to mean that there is no other way of producing atherosclerosis. What I mean to imply is that endogenous disturbances in the metabolism of cholesterol and/or fat play a considerable role in the development of human atherosclerosis, but without the presence of cholesterol in the diet, this endogenous disturbance may not occur. It is my opinion that cholesterol is the offending agent in atherosclerosis.

2. The answer is yes, since I have already said yes with some minor amendments to the first question.

3. My answer is no. There is no reason in our present state of knowledge to have the patient sharply restricted on cholesterol and fat as a preventative or as a cure, *except:*

(a) When a person is overweight he should have his diet reduced so as to approach the ideal weight. There is no doubt that obesity is definitely associated with an increased frequency of atherosclerosis. However, it would appear that the obesity itself is not the cause; it is the fact that the American and European diet is so rich in cholesterol that leads to the atherosclerosis tendency. Furthermore, in reducing, great care should be taken that there is no surplus of fat or cholesterol in the diet, since our work on chickens has shown that under such restricted diets the presence of any excess cholesterol is potentially more hazardous in developing atherosclerosis than on a normal caloric intake.

(b) When a patient has had two or more attacks of coronary insufficiency and/or myocardial infarction attributable to coronary atherosclerosis, and if that patient has a xanthomatotic tendency as revealed by the finding of his cholesterol level in the upper limits of normal, or above, then I believe I would recommend the reduction of cholesterol and fat in the diet. Otherwise, I would not, because I am a firm believer in the view that prohibitions should not be carelessly advocated until such time as it is clearly revealed that the prohibition has a great chance of being beneficial to the patient.

Ancel Keys, Ph.D.

1. The answer is a plain and simple *no*. The question would be more reasonably phrased to read: Has it been proved that human atherosclerosis *may* result—or results in some cases—from the ingestion of cholesterol and/or fat? But the answer would still be *no*.

2. The question must be more clearly defined. I think it more useful to try to answer several questions which, together, may cover the actual area of inquiry.

(a) If mankind stopped eating eggs, dairy products, meats and all visible fats, is it probable that all atherosclerosis would disappear?

The answer is *no*, but I believe atherosclerosis would become very rare.

(b) Is it probable that the development of human atherosclerosis is affected by the amount of cholesterol in any ordinary diets?

The answer is *no* except, possibly, in some rare individuals.

(c) Is it probable that the development of human atherosclerosis is affected by the amount of fats in any ordinary diets?

The answer is *yes*, but there are probably large differences among individuals.

3. The answer is that I would recommend a sharp reduction in all dietary fats without paying any special attention to the cholesterol content of the diet. I would allow the use of an ordinary amount of eggs and milk in cooking, the use of skim milk for cereals and as a beverage, a good daily serving of *lean* meat or fish, and a boiled or poached whole egg for Sunday; but no butter, cream, oleomargarine, salad oil, mayonnaise, fried foods, gravy, ice cream, chocolate, or pastries made with shortening. Periodic measurements of serum cholesterol may help to judge the severity with which such restrictions should be maintained.

John W. Gofman, M.D., Ph.D.

1. Atherosclerosis is associated, and very likely in an etiologic fashion, with the presence of certain special lipoprotein classes in the blood. There appears to be a metabolic derangement of lipid metabolism which leads to the appearance of higher levels of such lipopro-

teins in the blood of some individuals when compared with others. In the human, both sexes show low levels of such lipoproteins in childhood and early adulthood. In the later twenties the male surges ahead of the female and remains ahead statistically until approximately the age of 55. This metabolic derangement in lipid metabolism we regard as the underlying defect in the evolution of atherosclerosis. It may well be, from evidence reported elsewhere,* that a deficiency of heparin or a heparin-like substance is at the root of this lipoprotein metabolic defect. Dietary fat can raise the serum level of the atherogenic lipoproteins of the S_f 35–100 class acutely in many humans, and variably from individual to individual, depending upon the lipoprotein metabolism. Restriction of fats and cholesterol can depress the level of the atherogenic lipoproteins of the S_f 12–20 class and also of lipoproteins of the S_f 20–35 and S_f 35–100 classes. Yet there are individuals who can tolerate large quantities of dietary fat and cholesterol without showing abnormal lipoprotein patterns and, conversely, there are certain individuals who still show abnormal lipoprotein patterns in spite of dietary restriction of fat and cholesterol. Thus we would consider that the ingestion of fats and cholesterol, while most likely not responsible for the lipoprotein metabolic error and hence not the basic cause of atherosclerosis, can definitely contribute to atherosclerosis in many individuals because of the susceptibility of such individuals to the alteration of lipoprotein levels through diet.

2. This question has been partially answered in the answer to question one. We would reiterate here that, while the lipoprotein derangement which leads to atherosclerosis is probably not caused by dietary factors, it is exceedingly probable that dietary fat and cholesterol by unfavorably influencing the serum lipoprotein levels do contribute to the progression of atherosclerosis in a large fraction of the human population.

3. The vast majority of patients with clinical evidence of atherosclerosis will show elevations of the S_f 12–20, S_f 20–35, S_f 35–100 classes of lipoproteins. A large proportion of such patients will show improvement in the lipoprotein pattern on dietary restriction of fats and cholesterol, which improvement our evidence already indicates will lessen further clinical manifestations of atherosclerosis. Therefore,

* Page 66, reference 6.

the restriction of fat and cholesterol in the diet of such a patient has a very important place in the prophylactic and therapeutic armamentarium. It should be kept in mind, however, that because of the variability in ease of influencing lipoprotein levels by dietary measures certain patients will respond more favorably than others. We know at present of no way of predicting in a given patient whether or not the response to diet in the form of lipoprotein lowering will be large, intermediate or trivial. If a patient's lipoprotein levels can be studied ultracentrifugally, and it can be demonstrated that he responds to dietary restriction of fats and cholesterol with a significant lowering of lipoprotein levels, we would feel that there is ample reason to expect that atherogenesis can, in part at least, be suppressed by dietary means.

Experimental Atherosclerosis

By Louis N. Katz, M.D.

THIS PRESENTATION is concerned exclusively with one variety of arteriosclerosis, atherosclerosis. This subject delineation is not an arbitrary or artificial one. The term *arteriosclerosis* is a generic one. It refers to several distinct pathologic entities producing thickening of the vessel wall, embracing such entities as atherosclerosis, Mönckeberg's sclerosis, arteriolosclerosis, and hyperplastic arteriosclerosis. Awareness of this fact is absolutely essential for progress in this field. Recent research reinforces the conclusion that these are different entities. The attention of investigators is correctly focused today on the problem of the etiology and pathogenesis of *atherosclerosis*, since this is the lesion among the arterioscleroses which is overwhelmingly responsible for morbidity and mortality in man.

Until very recently atherosclerosis was a step-child problem of medical research commanding very limited resources of personnel, equipment, plant and money. This situation, only partially improved upon at present, is a consequence of several circumstances. Among them, one of the most important is a fundamentally erroneous concept developed in the medical profession itself—the senescence "theory" of the genesis of the arterioscleroses. This "theory" maintains that the arterioscleroses are inevitable results of physiologic aging processes. This "theory" likewise regards the specific entity atherosclerosis as such an unavoidable process of aging. The stagnating influence of this "theory" upon medical research has been overwhelming. It engendered an atmosphere of helplessness and hopelessness that was for many years a serious brake on all investigation.

This "theory" is a patently erroneous dogma. Certainly today overwhelming clinical evidence exists that atherosclerosis occurs in some very young people and is absent in some very old people. This indisputable evidence is alone sufficient to demonstrate that atherosclerosis cannot be an inevitable by-product of senescence. Rather, senescence and atherogenesis are two distinct and not necessarily related processes. Data from the experimental laboratory reinforce these conclusions of clinical research. Moreover, these data supply considerable support for the concept that atherogenesis is consequent upon an alteration in lipid metabolism, particularly in cholesterol metabolism.

It is upon the basis of this *cholesterol concept of atherogenesis* that fruitful research in this field is proceeding apace in a number of laboratories. The basic tenet of this concept may be simply stated: without an altered lipid-cholesterol metabolism little or no atherosclerosis will develop regardless of any other alterations in the arterial wall, including senescent changes. Obviously, if atherosclerotic lesions are the result—or even only in part the result—of altered lipid-cholesterol metabolism, then they are not inevitable. The whole foundation of the senescence theory is rendered untenable. The possibility, nay inevitability, presents itself that preventing or reversing the altered lipid-cholesterol metabolism will eliminate atherosclerosis. Thus, a hopeless situation is changed to one full of promise. Research in this field, by attacking the problem of the detailed interrelations between altered lipid-cholesterol metabolism and atherogenesis, can look forward to forging the scientific preconditions for eliminating atherosclerosis as a disease.

Evidence from Man

The cholesterol concept of atherosclerosis, the basis of almost all experimental work in this field at the present time, has an extensive foundation in clinical research. At least four sources have furnished supporting evidence for it: histopathology, biochemical pathology, ethnopathology and clinical pathology. A review of the extensive data from these sources is beyond the scope of this presentation. To summarize briefly the essential facts from these sources, histo- and chemicopathology early revealed that extensive lipid and cholesterol deposition is a hallmark of the atherosclerotic lesion. From the ethnopathologic viewpoint, comparative studies of vascular lesions among different peoples, including Costa Ricans, Okinawans, Chinese, Japanese, American and African Negroes, Eskimos and others, indicate that significant differences exist among peoples in incidence and severity of atherosclerosis. These differences appear to stem from culturally conditioned variations in nutrition and diet, rather than from racial, climatic or other influences. Specifically, a high correlation is frequently demonstrable between presence or absence of atherosclerosis and luxus or paucity of foods high in animal fat and cholesterol. Data accumulated in European countries during and after World Wars I and II lend further weight to the concept that there is a relationship of diet to atherogenesis. From these multiple studies the following tentative conservative conclusion appears justified: atherosclerosis is generally more frequent and severe in well nourished, particularly overnourished, people subsisting on diets rich in animal fat. Finally, from the clinicopathologic viewpoint, it is abundantly clear that in a number of disease states characterized by alterations in cholesterol metabolism and a prolonged hypercholesteremic phase, among them hypothyroidism, the nephrotic syndrome, essential familial xanthomatosis, biliary obstruction, and diabetes mel'itus, premature severe atherosclerosis is inordinately frequent. Moreover, evidence has recently accumulated indicating that patients with coronary atherosclerosis without gross hypercholesterolemia have subtle alterations in cholesterol metabolism and a "xanthomatous tendency." The suggestion, based on these data, of a close association between alterations in cholesterol metabolism and atherogenesis is further reinforced by the recent work of Gofman and his colleagues demonstrating abnormalities in circulating cholesterol-bearing lipoproteins in association with clinical atherosclerosis. This, in brief, constitutes the clinicopathologic background and foundation for experimental atherosclerosis.

Experimental Atherosclerosis

History

Experimental atherosclerosis was first successfully induced in animals in the period 1908 to 1912. Prior to that time, all experimental attempts to reproduce the atherosclerotic lesion of man had failed, although arterial lesions had been produced by a number of procedures in animals (such as treatment with drugs, pathogenic bacteria, toxins). However, the resultant changes in the vessels resembled the Mönckeberg type of human arteriosclerosis (medial calcinosis, senile arteriosclerosis), rather than atherosclerosis. In 1908 a group of investigators working in St. Petersburg studied the effects of various dietary regimens on vascular pathology. They observed that rabbits fed diets containing meat, milk or eggs developed atherosclerosis. It was soon demonstrated, particularly by Anitschkow, that the biochemical factor responsible for these lesions was cholesterol. Conclusive proof was advanced that this sterol was the atherogenic stimulus. Experimental atherosclerosis as a definitive field of research endeavor dates from these discoveries. It is noteworthy that to this day experimental atherosclerosis has not been successfully produced by any other means than cholesterol administration (except avian stilbestrol-induced atherosclerosis, a lesion secondary to endogenous endocrine-stimulated hypercholesteremic hyperlipemia).

The Chick as an Experimental Animal

About 10 years ago this department became interested in experimental atherosclerosis. Our studies were carried on in the past decade principally in the chick. Our choice of this experimental animal was not fortuitous. Rather, it was based on a purposeful attempt to proceed along lines obviating criticisms leveled by many at the use of the rabbit for such atherosclerosis research. The rabbit is a herbivorous species not normally ingesting cholesterol. Moreover, on its usual diet it does not naturally develop vascular lesions of the atherosclerotic variety. Finally, until the last decade experimentalists had experienced only limited and indifferent success in attempts to induce gross atherosclerotic lesions by cholesterol feeding in species other than the rabbit. All these facts led many workers to question seriously the relevance of cholesterol-induced atherosclerosis in the rabbit for an understanding of the pathogenesis of the human disease. It was upon this basis that we sought to find a more suitable experimental animal. The chick was finally selected after a careful survey of the extant literature.

The chick, like man, is omnivorous, and develops atherosclerotic lesions of the great vessels spontaneously. In early studies it was quickly demonstrated that cholesterol feeding led to hypercholesteremia and eventually to atherogenesis in chicks. Such cholesterol-fed birds had gross atherosclerosis not only of the aorta, but also of the major systemic vessels, including the coronary arteries. These cholesterol-induced lesions were readily distinguishable from spontaneous lesions. Further, cholesterol was readily shown to be the decisive atherogenic stimulus in chicks, as in rabbits.

These initial studies demonstrated that the chick is of unique utility in offering two types of lesions for experimental study, the spontaneous and the cholesterol-induced. In 1946 the horizon and methodology of experimental atherosclerosis in the chick were further broadened. In that year Chaikoff and his associates showed that atherosclerosis occurred in cockerels having a prolonged endogenous hyperlipemia induced by implantation of estrogenic material. Horlick and Katz confirmed this finding and extended it by demonstrating that the lesions in stilbestrol-treated chicks were definitely not of the spontaneous type. Thus, a third experimental lesion in chicks became available for study. This avian species possesses, then, a unique versatility which further enhances its utility in atherosclerosis research.

Morphology of Atherosclerosis in the Chick

In several publications from this department, a detailed description has been given of the morphology of spontaneous, cholesterol-induced and stilbestrol-induced atherosclerosis in cockerels. A general review of the pathology of these lesions is beyond the scope of this presentation. However, several specific points may be noted: (1) Detailed microscopic studies indicate that throughout the arterial tree of stilbestrol-treated or cholesterol-fed chicks the primary lesion of experimental atherosclerosis is the foam cell intimal cushion. This lesion, so-called pure atheroma, is almost certainly the first stage of atherogenesis. The morphologic patterns of more advanced lesions are apparently the result of evolutionary pathologic processes secondary to atheroma. (2) It is possible by prolonged cholesterol feeding to induce in chicks the spectrum of atherosclerotic changes seen in human lesions including foam cell plaques, necrosis and atheromatous abscesses, fibrosis and hyalinization, calcification and cartilaginous-osseous metaplasia. Ulceration of atherosclerotic plaques with thrombus formation is the only lesion seen in man that has not been observed in cholesterol-fed chicks. (3) Cholesterol feeding apparently aggravates and intensifies spontaneous lesions. It would appear that the fibrotic spontaneous lesion is a site of predilection for cholesterol and lipid deposition, with subsequent evolutionary atherosclerotic changes. (4) Despite persistent dogma to the contrary, our experiments conclusively demonstrate that atherosclerotic lesions are reversible. (These findings are in accord with accumulated observations in man and rabbit.) Horlick and Katz demonstrated in the cholesterol-fed chick that in the weeks following cessation of cholesterol feeding, definite regression and healing of cholesterol-induced lesions occurred. Previously existing moderately severe atheromatous lesions apparently completely healed and disappeared. More advanced lesions underwent partial resolution and evolution.

The question has been repeatedly posed: are experimental and human lesions morphologically similar? Even the most severe critics of the cholesterol concept of atherosclerosis cannot fail to note the conspicuous similarities between cholesterol-induced lesions—whether in rabbit, dog or chick—and the lesions seen in man. Taking into consideration the anatomic differences among the various species in architecture of the great vessels, the similarities between experimental cholesterol-induced and human lesions are indeed remarkable. That this resemblance is more than fortuitous is further emphasized by the fact that such lesions have not been produced experimentally by any other means.

Amount and Duration of Cholesterol Feeding

Our initial experiments on chick atherosclerosis placed us in a position to study possible exogenous and endogenous factors influencing the three types of avian lesions. However, preliminary to such investigations it became essential to quantitate the relation of the amount and duration of cholesterol feeding to the degree of hypercholesterolemia and to the incidence and severity of atherosclerosis. Toward this end several experiments were accomplished utilizing various levels of cholesterol in the diet and various feeding periods.

Further, in order to permit quantitative evaluation of lesions, a system for gross grading of aortas for atherosclerosis was devised. This grading method, like others, is undoubtedly empiric and subjective. However, when employed with necessary precautions to guarantee treating all specimens as unknowns, it yields reliable information as to both incidence and severity of lesions. Hence it makes possible quantitation of pathologic data. By means of this grading method a general relationship is readily demonstrable between atherogenesis (incidence and severity of lesions) and cholesterol ingestion (amount and duration of sterol feeding). Thus with ranges of dietary cholesterol between 0.25 and 2.0 per cent (plus 5 per cent cottonseed oil), biochemical and pathologic alterations are quantitatively parallel. This is true both with chicks placed on experimental diets at 4 to 6 weeks of age and when 1 day old. In the course of these studies an additional basic methodologic principle became clear: In order to assess accurately the influence of various factors on experimental atherosclerosis, studies must be controlled with respect to each and every one of the following factors—age, sex, initial weight, feed intake, final weight and (at least in the chick) season. Attention to these elements in experiments on atherosclerosis insures a high degree of reliable quantitation in results.

Undernutrition and Overnutrition

Based on these studies it became possible to determine the influence of various factors on experimental atherosclerosis. The influence of one such factor, undernutrition, was explored in several experiments. In an early experiment, Dauber and Katz demonstrated that underfeeding per se (without cholesterol supplement in the diet) failed to induce lesions of the cholesterol type or to influence spontaneous atherogenesis. Subsequently, Rodbard and co-workers analyzed the effects of undernutrition on cholesterol-induced lesions. In one series of experiments chicks were fed mash containing either 0.25 per cent cholesterol plus 5 per cent oil or 2 per cent cholesterol. At each dietary level, one group of birds was permitted to eat ad libitum, another was given only 60 to 70 per cent as much mash. Chicks on this reduced dietary intake received less cholesterol than the controls given the same mash ad libitum. Nevertheless the semi-starved birds tended to have a more severe hypercholesteremia than the controls. At the conclusion of the experiment incidence and severity of atherosclerosis in the undernourished cockerels were as great as or greater than in the control birds on an unrestricted diet of similar composition. Apparently the underfed birds were not readily able either to draw upon the elevated plasma lipids as a source of calories or to dispose of the exogenous cholesterol load. Thus it may be concluded that cholesterol remains an atherogenic stimulus regardless of the level of over-all caloric intake. It may be further suggested that in Europeans and Americans, where a definitive correlation has been shown between obesity and intensified atherogenesis, this influence of obesity may be attributable to the associated increased intake of specific atherogenic material, that is, cholesterol.

In another series of experiments, Rodbard and co-workers approached the same general problem somewhat differently; chicks were fed cholesterol diets during repeated short intervals. During interim periods (one to five days in duration), they were either starved or fed plain mash. A third group subsisted on the cholesterol diet continuously. The cholesterol-fed birds, starved during alternate periods, developed marked hypercholesteremia and atherosclerosis, resembling the findings in cockerels on a continuous cholesterol mash diet. In contrast, chicks alternating between cholesterol diet and regular mash exhibited only slight hypercholesteremia and atherosclerosis. Thus intermittent periods of starvation apparently hindered, rather than facilitated, the disposal of exogenous cholesterol load, whereas intermittent periods of regular mash facilitated such disposal. Over-all adequate intake of a balanced diet apparently made a key contribution to preventing dietary induced hypercholesteremia and atherosclerosis. Whether this effect is mediated by dietary or endocrine factors, or both, remains to be elucidated. These findings suggest the possibility that in man the effects of exogenous cholesterol on cholesteremia and atherogenesis may be at least in part regulated by over-all nutritional status.

In contrast to these experimental studies on semistarvation, only limited observations are available on the effects of overfeeding on experimental atherogenesis. To our knowledge only one report in the literature deals with this problem. Wolffe and associates indicate that force fed geese exhibit an increased incidence of both spontaneous and cholesterol-induced atherosclerosis. Evaluation of these findings awaits publication of the complete data. Since obesity, the level of food intake in general, and cholesterol intake in particular have all been implicated as important factors in human atherogenesis, further experimental studies are indicated on excessive dietary intake and atherosclerosis.

Neutral Fat in Diet

Among other exogenous factors possibly influencing atherogenesis, neutral fat intake has been studied experimentally by us. In initial experiments, Dauber and Katz observed no effect of 20 per cent cottonseed oil diets on lipemia or spontaneous atherogenesis in chicks. More recently Stamler and co-workers extended these observations to chicks fed mash supplemented with 5 per cent cottonseed oil. Here again normal plasma lipid patterns were observed, no effect on spontaneous atherogenesis was noted, and no lesions of the cholesterol-induced variety supervened.

These experiments cannot be interpreted as indicating that neutral fat ingestion is not a factor in human atherogenesis. Clinically, neutral fat and cholesterol ingestion are almost invariably combined—in contrast to the foregoing experiments. Considerable evidence exists that under such circumstances triglyceride influences cholesterol metabolism. Moreover, a recent experiment in our laboratory also indicates that under certain circumstances neutral fat ingestion affects cholesterol metabolism and atherogenesis in the chick. Briefly, Stamler and associates demonstrated that depancreatized chicks respond differently to cholesterol feeding, depending on the presence or absence of cottonseed oil in the mash.

Cholesterol-Free and Fat-Poor Diet

In other studies on exogenous factors, Horlick and his colleagues analyzed the effects of a specially prepared defatted mash on both spontaneous and stilbestrol-induced atherosclerosis in cockerels. They also investigated the influence of such a low fat, cholesterol-free mash on regression of cholesterol-induced atherosclerosis occurring upon cessation of cholesterol feeding. In the first study, chicks receiving defatted mash developed spontaneous aorta lesions later than birds subsisting on regular mash; these lesions were less extensive and severe. However, lesions were present. Hence the defatted mash diet failed to eliminate spontaneous arteriosclerosis in the chicks although it may have retarded this pathologic process. Apparently an exogenous source of lipid and cholesterol is not essential for spontaneous arterio- sclerosis in the chick. If plasma lipids play a key role in such spontane- ous arteriosclerosis, endogenous sources cont nue to make available sufficient lipids for this process. It might appear from these experi- ments that the spontaneous lesions produced are primarily arterio- sclerotic and only secondarily atherosclerotic.

In a second experiment, Horlick and Katz observed that a defatted mash was without significant effect on the endogenous hyperlipemia and hypercholesteremia induced by stilbestrol implantation in cockerels. Stilbestrol-induced atherogenesis developed concomitant with the hypercholesteremia in these estrogen-treated birds fed a de- fatted mash.

In a third study with defatted mash, the influence of this diet on regression of cholesterol-induced lesions was analyzed by Horlick and Katz in chicks rendered atherosclerotic by a prolonged period of cholesterol feeding. The specially prepared defatted mash was no more valuable in effecting the regression of atherosclerotic lesion than the regular chick starter mash.

The fact that spontaneous arteriosclerotic lesions occur with choles- terol-free, fat-poor diet, and that this diet had no obvious effect in eliminating the endogenously induced lesions casts some doubt on the view that *low fat diets in man* exert any marked influence on athero- sclerosis. The conclusive proof for such a view must still be forth- coming. It is not at present available. It seems pertinent to suggest that in the present state of knowledge, use of low fat, low cholesterol diets in man would appear justified only (a) in cases with abnormally high cholesterol blood levels and (b) in patients with more than one episode of recent myocardial infarction, who have blood cholesterol levels at the upper limits of normal or above normal. Furthermore, the dietary restriction under such circumstances must be drastic; for example, a diet of 25 to 50 Gm. of fat per day must be rigidly adhered to, and it must be persisted in for long periods of time. The obvious difficulties of pursuing such a program and the inconclusiveness of the results obtained should make one hesitant to undertake widespread use of such dietary restraints until the controversy concerning the effects is settled conclusively one way or the other.

Lipotropic Factors

Among dietary factors possibly influencing human and experimental atherosclerosis, greatest attention has focused on lipotropic factors. Until recently their value was not clear, since contradictory findings were reported concerning the effects of these factors. This confusion has been eliminated in the last year or two. Experiments in chick, dog and rabbit yielding negative results are particularly decisive in indicating that at least choline is of no value in the prophylaxis or therapy of atherosclerosis. In this laboratory Stamler and co-workers studied the possible prophylactic influences of choline and inositol in spontaneous, cholesterol-induced and stilbestrol-induced atherosclerosis in cockerels. In the studies of lipotropic factors in cholesterol-induced atherosclerosis, the effects of 1 per cent choline plus 1 per cent inositol were determined in birds fed three different concentrations of dietary cholesterol, 0.25, 0.5 and 2 per cent. In studies continuing from 15 to 35 weeks all experimental regimens were well tolerated; normal feed intakes and rates of weight gain were recorded throughout. All cholesterol diets produced hypercholesteremia and hyperlipemia of varying degrees, hypercholesteremia being the principal alteration in the plasma lipid pattern. Phospholipids rose, but disproportionately less than cholesterol so the plasma total cholesterol–lipid phosphorus (C/P) ratio increased significantly. At all levels of cholesterol feeding 1 per cent choline plus 1 per cent inositol failed consistently to lower hypercholesteremia and hyperlipemia. The lipotropic factors were without effect in ameliorating the minimal hypercholesteremia consequent upon feeding 0.25 per cent cholesterol mash. The data indicate that during the initial weeks of the experiment addition of lipotropic factors to the diet actually aggravated hypercholesteremia. The exhibition of the phospholipid precursors choline and inositol failed significantly to elevate plasma phospholipid levels sufficiently or to correct the abnormally high plasma total cholesterol–lipid phosphorus ratios. Choline and inositol had only a limited incomplete lipotropic effect on cholesterol-induced hepatic lipidosis and completely failed to influence the lipidosis in other organs, including the aorta. Similarly the lipotropic factors failed to reduce the incidence or severity of cholesterol-induced lesions in either the thoracic or abdominal aorta.

In the companion experiments, Stamler and co-workers demonstrated that the lipotropic factors were also without significant effect on the hyperlipemia of stilbestrol administration and on either stilbestrol-induced or spontaneous atherogenesis. Recent reports of carefully controlled studies by Firstbrook and Davidson and associates similarly indicate that choline is ineffective as a prophylactic or therapeutic agent against cholesterol-induced atherosclerosis in rabbits and dogs. Insofar as studies in man are concerned, adequately controlled clinical data are lacking; the efficacy of lipotropic factors in the prophylaxis or therapy of human atherosclerosis has not been demonstrated. Hence we deem it necessary to emphasize that neither clinical nor experimental foundations are present to justify the widespread prescription of costly preparations of lipotropic factors for human atherosclerosis. Such procedure merits condemnation on both scientific and socioeconomic grounds.

Aluminum Hydroxide Gel

Since cholesterol undergoes an enterohematohepatic circulation, the possibility presents itself that the intestinal disposal of cholesterol might be enhanced, plasma cholesterol levels thereby lowered, and atherogenesis retarded. Rodbard and his colleagues have been carrying out experiments on this problem in our laboratory. Utilizing a specially prepared aluminum hydroxide gel, it has been possible to decrease hypercholesteremia and atherogenesis in cholesterol-fed cockerels. This problem is under further study in our laboratory at the present time.

Cholesterol–Phospholipid Ratio

A number of recent investigators have brought forward evidence from studies on man suggesting that the plasma cholesterol–phospholipid (C/P) ratio may be a key factor in atherogenesis. Since cholesterol-induced atherosclerosis in rabbit, chick and dog is uniformly associated with a disturbed lipid pattern characterized by hypercholesteremia, altered cholesterol–phospholipid ratios and chylomicronemia the question arises: is the hypercholesteremia per se or the altered cholesterol–phospholipid ratio the decisive factor in atherogenesis? Can atherogenesis occur without an elevated cholesterol–phospholipid ratio?

Several studies in our laboratory bear upon this problem of cholesterol–phospholipid ratios and atherogenesis. First, it is noteworthy that estrogen-treated chicks, unlike cholesterol-fed birds, exhibit a plasma lipid pattern characterized by hyperphospholipemia in excess of hypercholesteremia, with a resultant lowering of the plasma cholesterol–phospholipid ratio. Aortic atherosclerosis eventually supervenes in birds subjected to prolonged estrogen treatment. Under these experimental conditions a fall in the cholesterol–phospholipid ratio prevents neither plasma lactescence nor aortic atherosclerosis.

In another experiment Stamler and Katz attempted to correlate plasma biochemical data and postmortem pathologic findings in individual chicks fed 0.25 per cent cholesterol mash for 35 weeks, beginning at 5 weeks of age. Analysis of these data reveal a close correlation between the level of hypercholesteremia and aortic atherogenesis in individual birds. In contrast, there was no correlation between presence or absence of induced lesions in the aorta and degree of elevation of the plasma cholesterol–phospholipid ratio. Thus, this experiment demonstrated a lack of correlation between plasma cholesterol–phospholipid ratios and aortic atherogenesis, together with a positive correlation between plasma cholesterol levels and aortic lesions.

Although these experiments indicate that cholesterol–phospholipid ratios are not decisive factors for aorta atherogenesis, recent studies by Pick and associates in our laboratory indicate that cholesterol–phospholipid ratios and *coronary* atherogenesis may be closely interrelated. Thus, estrogen exhibition to cholesterol-fed chicks results in suppression of coronary atherogenesis. Concomitantly, the ratios are depressed to or toward normal, despite persistent cholesterol-induced hypercholesterolemia.

This finding of prophylactic inhibition of coronary atherosclerosis by estrogens may be a significant lead concerning the mechanism of the well known sex differential in human susceptibility to coronary atherosclerosis. Further, since cholesterol-fed chicks are not protected against aorta atherosclerosis by estrogens, but are protected against coronary lesions, it would appear that atherogenesis proceeds according to different biologic laws in different vascular beds. Evidence is extant indicating a similar phenomenon in man. Hence, investigation of experimental atherosclerosis should not be confined to aorta lesions, lest significant findings in such important beds as the coronary and cerebral be entirely overlooked.

Thyroid

In addition to the foregoing studies, this department has carried on a number of experiments on the influences of various endogenous factors upon experimental atherogenesis. Among such factors studied to date, thyroid hormone has been found to be far and away the most effective agent influencing experimental atherogenesis. In an initial study in this laboratory, Dauber and associates demonstrated that desiccated thyroid significantly depressed the hypercholesteremia of birds given diets supplemented with 0.5 to 2.0 per cent cholesterol plus 20 per cent cottonseed oil. In accordance with these plasma lipid patterns thyroid hormone significantly decreased the incidence and severity of cholesterol-induced atherosclerosis. In a subsequent study, Stamler and co-workers extended these observations to stilbestrol-induced atherosclerosis in cockerels. Although desiccated thyroid only temporarily depressed the hyperlipemia of chronic stilbestrol administration, it was remarkably effective in reducing the incidence and severity of lesions in the aorta.

The mechanism or mechanisms of this effect of thyroid hormone on atherosclerosis remain obscure. Various hypotheses have been advanced by different investigators, among them that thyroid exerts its effect directly on cholesterol metabolism, reducing the hypercholesteremic stimulus to atherogenesis; that thyroid hormone affects the tissue accumulation of cholesterol; that thyroid hormone alters vascular permeability. Unfortunately, little is known concerning the mechanisms whereby thyroid affects lipid metabolism. Recent studies with radioactive tracers indicate that thyroid influences the hepatic degradation of the lipids, effecting lipid depletion.

In one of our studies Stamler and his colleagues undertook to determine whether the influence of thyroid hormone on lipids and atherosclerosis is a simple by-product of induced hypermetabolism. A comparison was made of the effect of desiccated thyroid and of the hypermetabolism-inducing drug dinitrophenol on plasma and tissue lipids and atherogenesis in cholesterol-fed chicks. Despite the similar hypermetabolism-inducing potential of thyroid and dinitrophenol, markedly different effects of the two substances were observed in these cholesterol-fed birds. Unlike the birds given thyroid hormone, the dinitrophenol-fed animals failed to exhibit a depression of either hypercholesteremia or atherogenesis. This experiment therefore suggests that the effects of thyroid hormone on lipid metabolism and atherogenesis cannot be attributed solely to any generalized non-specific increase in energy exchange it induces. Rather than being non-specific by-products of increased metabolic rate, these actions of thyroid on cholesterol metabolism would appear to be effected via specific metabolic reactions involving hormone and lipids—reactions whose pathways are today obscure.

Pancreas

In view of the increased incidence and severity of atherosclerosis in clinical diabetes, the role of the pancreas (as well as the other endocrine glands involved in the pathogenesis of diabetes) in experimental atherosclerosis merits considerable attention. Until recently, experimental work on this aspect of atherosclerosis was very limited in scope. A few reports indicate that atherosclerotic lesions eventually develop in chronic diabetic dogs, particularly in completely depancreatized insulin-maintained animals subsisting on a diet of moderate to high fat content without supplementary raw pancreas or lipotropic factor. Experimental work on these problems in the rat, a species which to date has proved to be particularly resistant to cholesterol-induced atherosclerosis, has been even more limited. In this and other departments no success has been obtained in efforts to induce atherosclerosis by cholesterol feeding in alloxan diabetic rats. In rabbits, several workers report cataracts, but no atherosclerosis, following long-standing alloxan diabetes. When alloxan diabetes is combined with cholesterol feeding, the unexpected observation was made that atherogenesis tended to be retarded. Duff and Paine attributed this finding to the interrelations between cholesterol and phospholipid (normal C/P ratios) in such animals. It has also been suggested that this inhibitory phenomenon may be due to undernutrition and emaciation in alloxan diabetic rabbits.

It may be noted at this point that the study of the role of lipotropic factors in experimental atherosclerosis has its roots in the original observations that totally depancreatized, insulin-treated dogs can be chronically maintained only if fed a supplement of raw pancreas or its decisive lipotropic factors, lecithin or choline. Hence, in a certain sense the studies on lipotropic factors (which, as already noted, have yielded negative results) are an aspect of the problem of the role of the pancreas in experimental atherosclerosis.

In our laboratory, we have studied this over-all problem in chicks. This animal is readily amenable to total pancreatectomy or alloxanization. In an initial study, Stamler and co-workers determined the effect of pancreatectomy on plasma and tissue lipids and on the three types of chick atherosclerosis. In totally depancreatized cockerels fed a regular mash, free of cholesterol or other supplements, both plasma lipid and carbohydrate level are within normal limits. These birds exhibit no overt signs of metabolic disturbance. Lesions of the induced variety do not develop, although these chicks exhibit a tendency to intensified spontaneous arteriosclerosis. Stilbestrol-treated, depancreatized birds also exhibit a plasma lipid pattern essentially similar to that of their unoperated controls.

When a supplement of cholesterol and cottonseed oil is added to the mash of depancreatized cockerels, a plasma lipid pattern emerges that is significantly different quantitatively from that of their paired controls. They consistently exhibit a far more severe hypercholesteremia; this is accompanied by intensified atherogenesis. In contrast, when depancreatized chicks are fed a mash containing cholesterol, but devoid of a cottonseed oil supplement, they exhibit a plasma lipid pattern essentially similar to their unoperated paired controls on a similar diet. Thus, the addition of neutral fat to the diet apparently plays a decisive role in the development of an inordinate hypercholesteremia in pancreatectomized cholesterol-fed chicks. Since depancreatized cockerels fed a cholesterol–cottonseed oil mash exhibit a response different from their paired controls, it may be concluded that this dietary regimen has brought out subtle defects of lipid metabolism in these birds. Similarly, it is possible to bring out subtle defects in carbohydrate metabolism. Although chronically depancreatized chicks on regular diet exhibit gross derangement in neither plasma lipid nor glucose level, the administration of adrenocortical extract to such birds results in a marked hyperglycemia, far in excess of that seen in unoperated controls, and reaching levels well into the severe diabetic range.

These two experiments indicate that in the chick, as in man, the pancreas apparently plays an important role in the metabolism of both the lipids and carbohydrates. This biologic similarity emerges despite initial data indicating that pancreatic deficiency has different effects on metabolism in chick and man. Our findings suggest that these apparent differences between man and chick are not necessarily qualitative ones, but rather at least in part quantitative. The relationships of both lipid and carbohydrate metabolic effects to atherogenesis in the chick are under further investigation in this laboratory.

Hypertension

In view of the frequent clinical observation that hypertension is associated with intensified atherogenesis in man, we undertook to study the interrelationship between these two pathologic processes in the experimental animal. The demonstration by Lenel and associates in our laboratory that salt feeding induces a significant chronic rise in blood pressure in chicks made it possible to carry on such experiments. In an initial study, Stamler and Katz compared atherogenesis in salt hypertensive and normotensive cockerels subsisting on a diet of regular mash *without* a cholesterol supplement. The experimental regimens had no effect on plasma cholesterol concentration. Despite a significant elevation of blood pressure in the salt-treated animals, no gross lesions of the induced type were observed, nor was there any clear-cut intensification of spontaneous lesions. Thus, salt hypertension had little or no effect in grossly intensifying *spontaneous* arteriosclerosis in cockerels.

In a subsequent study, Stamler and co-workers analyzed the effect of another type of hypertension on atherogenesis in chicks subsisting on plain mash: namely, desoxycorticosterone acetate (DCA)–salt hypertension. Here again, in the absence of a supplement of cholesterol in the diet, no lesions of the induced type were observed, nor was there intensification of *spontaneous* lesions. It would appear that in the presence of consistent normocholesteremia, hypertension is ineffective as an atherogenic stimulus, both with respect to causing the appearance of induced lesions and with respect to intensifying spontaneous lesions. This finding is in accord with observations in this and other laboratories with several other species, including rabbit, dog, sheep and goat.

In contrast to such negative results, desoxycorticosterone-salt hypertension did intensify cholesterol-induced atherogenesis in cholesterol-fed cockerels. This observation, too, is consistent with the findings of other workers utilizing rabbits and dogs; namely, that hypertension intensifies atherogenesis when accompanied by a cholesterol diet. The mechanism of this effect remains obscure. Regardless of mechanism, however, the facts available from these experiments support the view enunciated by several investigators: cholesterol is the decisive factor in the pathogenesis of atherosclerosis, whereas hypertension acts rather as an intensifying agent, exerting this effect when the lipid metabolic situation favors atherogenesis.

Vascular Damage

Some workers attribute the effect of hypertension on atherosclerosis to a vascular damage presumably caused by hyperpiesis. Fundamental to such a concept is the problem: is pre-existent vascular damage a prerequisite for lipid deposition and atherogenesis? Numerous attempts were made to clarify this problem experimentally. A host of noxious agents were tested for atherogenic effect, including bacteria, toxins, drugs, hormones, mechanical and thermal trauma. Although various lesions were experimentally produced by these methods, atherosclerosis was never produced. Thus it would appear that in the absence of an essential lipid metabolic alteration, vascular damage, per se, is ineffective as an atherogenic stimulus. On the other hand, experimental and clinical data from a number of sources indicate that foci of vascular damage are sites of predilection for deposition of atherogenic material, provided the necessary lipid metabolic alteration is present.

Some of the experiments in our laboratory bear upon this problem. In a recent study by Rodbard and his colleagues, 1 day old cockerels were placed on a diet of chick starter mash supplemented with 2 per cent cholesterol plus 5 per cent cottonseed oil. Weekly sacrifice of birds on this regimen revealed gross cholesterol-induced lesions of the aorta in birds as young as 5 weeks of age. It is apparent that these chicks had juvenile arterial tissue. Their vascular wall had not yet been subject to necrobiotic senescent alterations. Moreover, during their brief 5 weeks in the laboratory there was no indication in these healthy birds of the operation of pathologic stimuli noxious to the vessel wall other than the hyperlipemia itself. The occurrence of significant gross atherosclerosis in these cockerels suggests, therefore, that atherogenesis may proceed solely on the basis of deranged lipid metabolism, provided this is severe enough in degree and duration. On the other hand, Schlichter and associates have shown in dogs that vascular damage to the outer third or half of the aorta produced by cauterization focally alters the arterial wall, so that the subjacent intima becomes a site of predilection for deposition of administered atherogenic material (cholesterol). These and supplementary data of a similar nature from other laboratories lead us to agree with Anitschkow's original concept, advanced many years ago, that cholesterol may be a *primary* atherogenic stimulus. We are also in accord with his further concept that vascular damage may play a role in the arterial deposition of lipids. These ideas, called the "combined theory" by Anitschkow, recognize that a number of different factors are involved in the pathogenesis of atherosclerosis; they also recognize the key role of the lipids in atherogenesis, whereby a severe enough derangement of lipid metabolism may result in atherogenesis in previously normal vessels; they further recognize that with less marked derangements in cholesterol metabolism, atherogenesis may still proceed, particularly in sites of predilection produced by previous vascular damage.

Pituitary and Adrenals

In connection with these concepts of the role of vascular damage in the pathogenesis of atherosclerosis, considerable attention has recently been focused upon the influence of the adrenal steroids, particularly since several workers have demonstrated vascular injury in animals chronically treated with desoxycorticosterone acetate and other corticoids. This problem assumes further importance in view of the fact that clinical endocrine disorders characterized by excessive secretion of adrenal steroids (e.g., Cushing's syndrome) are associated with intensified atherogenesis. Introduction into clinical therapeutics of adrenocorticotropic hormone (ACTH) and cortisone further highlights the need to investigate the possibility that steroids may be atherogenic, particularly since chronic treatment with cortisone may result in a significant rise in the plasma cholesterol concentration of man. Finally we should take note of the fact that the adrenal cortex plays an active part in sterol metabolism as is indicated by their high concentration of cholesterol, their ability readily to discharge cholesterol, to synthesize cholesterol, and to accumulate ingested cholesterol.

We have already briefly referred to the results of our studies on athero-genesis in desoxycorticosterone acetate-salt treated birds. Although moderate hyperpiesis supervened, no effect was observed on spontane-ous lesions. However, cholesterol-induced atherogenesis tended to be moderately intensified. A more recent experiment by Stamler and associates further demonstrated that cortisone intensified aorta and coronary atherogenesis in cholesterol-fed chicks, although this steroid did not alter blood pressure or plasma lipid levels. Obviously these are not exhaustive experiments on the pituitary-adrenocortical axis and atherogenesis. The possible influences of other glycocorticoids remain to be explored. Such studies are currently in progress in this labora-tory. Also in need of further study are the complex interrelationships between the hypothalamic-pituitary-adrenocortical system and the other endocrines.

Aging

Among the endogenous factors possibly influencing atherogenesis, careful consideration must be given to the problem of age. A recent study by Rodbard and associates in our laboratory yielded significant findings concerning the influence of age on cholesteremia and athero-genesis. These workers recorded age-associated variations in level of cholesteremia in cockerels on a diet of constant cholesterol content. Thus, during the first seven weeks of life, birds on a diet containing 2 per cent cholesterol plus 5 per cent cottonseed oil exhibited a choles-teremia in the range of 200 to 500 mg. per 100 cc. At about the eighth week, this cholesteremia increased spontaneously to a level of 800 to 900 mg. per 100 cc., although no change was instituted in the experi-mental regimen. This new high level of cholesteremia tended to main-tain itself during the next 12 weeks. At about the twentieth week of age, with the same diet continuing, there was a secondary fall of the plasma cholesterol level to about 300 to 500 mg. per 100 cc. In accord with these plasma lipid findings, atherogenesis during the first seven weeks of life was slight, whereas it proceeded rapidly after the eighth week. This experiment indicates that endogenous factors varying with age influence the response of chicks to a diet containing cholesterol. These endogenous factors, conditioned by and varying with age, in-fluence both cholesterol metabolism and atherogenesis. Preliminary evidence suggests that hormonal factors may play a key role in this varying pattern of endogenous control of cholesterol metabolism.

Gonads

Among other endogenous factors possibly influencing atherogenesis, attention must be focused upon the role of the gonads, particularly in view of the conspicuous sex difference in the incidence of coronary disease in human beings. Experimental work on the gonads and atherogenesis has been limited. An extensive investigation of this problem is currently in progress in our laboratory. As already indicated, estrogens have been shown to inhibit coronary lesions in cholesterol-fed cockerels. A few reports are extant of experiments in the rabbit. These observations are patently incomplete and require supplementation by more extensive investigation.

Species Differences

Among the problems that emerge in the course of studying atherosclerosis experimentally, perhaps the most intriguing is the one of species differences in susceptibility to lesions. Man, the chick and the duck develop atherosclerosis "spontaneously." The dog and the rabbit rarely do. Experimentally it is easy to produce gross atherosclerosis in rabbits or chicks. It is more difficult in guinea pigs, hamsters and ducks. It is still more difficult in dogs. To date it has proved impossible consistently to produce gross atherosclerosis in rats. Why these species differences in atherogenesis? In our laboratory Schlichter has suggested that they may depend on species variability in the adequacy of the vasa vasorum of the large arteries. On the other hand, considerable evidence exists indicating that species differences in atherogenesis may depend on species variability in lipid metabolism. Studies by Horlick and co-workers in our department, utilizing the intravenous cholesterol tolerance technic, suggest that such variations exist. Thus the disappearance time of intravenously injected cholesterol is not the same in three species investigated to date. For proportional amounts of cholesterol the disappearance time in the rabbit is about 72 hours, in the chick 24 hours, in the rat 12 hours. Recent ultracentrifuge and isotope studies also demonstrate species differences in lipoprotein and cholesterol metabolism. Moreover there are well-known marked species differences in the cholesteremic response to orally ingested cholesterol. In general, ease of hypercholesteremia production and ease of atherosclerosis production parallel each other among the various species.

Finally, it is noteworthy that only in the rabbit and chick (and perhaps in man) can atherosclerosis be produced with but slight hypercholesteremia, resulting from chronic cholesterol ingestion by these experimental animals. Undoubtedly further research will clarify the reasons for the foregoing species differences in lipid metabolism and atherogenesis. Undoubtedly such advances will be fruitful contributions to the ultimate solution of the whole atherosclerosis problem.

Minimal Cholesteremia

In the foregoing sections, we have briefly reviewed the experimental work of our department on atherosclerosis. As indicated, in many of our experiments the dosage of cholesterol utilized resulted in marked hypercholesteremia and organ lipidosis, as well as atherosclerosis. The criticism has been frequently advanced that lesions occurring under such circumstances are fundamentally different from those seen in most human beings (excepting those with gross xanthomatosis), since atherosclerosis frequently occurs in people with presumably normal or near normal plasma and tissue cholesterol concentrations. In view of this frequently advanced criticism, Stamler and associates undertook two long-term experiments to explore this problem further, particularly in an effort to produce cholesterol-induced atherosclerosis in the chick with minimal concomitant hypercholesteremia and organ lipidosis. It was found that a diet of 0.25 per cent cholesterol mash induces a minimal hypercholesteremia and organ lipidosis in chicks. Maintaining chicks on this diet for periods beyond 15 to 20 weeks had a profound effect on atherogenesis, in the presence of minimal changes in plasma and tissue lipid concentrations. A high incidence was found of moderately severe gross atherosclerosis of the cholesterol-induced type in the thoracic aorta. These experiments demonstrated clearly that significant cholesterol-induced atherogenesis proceeds in chicks fed a dietary level of sterol inducing little or no hypercholesteremia and organ lipidosis. These findings in the chick are in accord with previous experimental work in the rabbit.

When they are evaluated in relation to the latest data on man, these observations assume particular significance. Thus, today a mass of data exists demonstrating that a "xanthomatous tendency" (minimal hypercholesteremia) prevails in many people who are victimized by atherosclerosis. Moreover, considerable evidence is available indicating that cholesterol "input loads" (the quantity of ingested cholesterol per unit time that the body must absorb, transport, metabolize, turn over and excrete) influences atherogenesis in man. This conclusion is reinforced by the recent studies of Gofman indicating that diet may vary the concentration of various classes and species of plasma cholesterol-bearing lipoprotein molecules including classes and species tentatively implicated in the pathogenesis of atherosclerosis.

Conclusion

In conclusion, we may reiterate that a basic proposition has been the foundation of the work of this department on experimental atherosclerosis. The essence of this proposition is that altered cholesterol metabolism plays a key role in human atherogenesis. The corollary of this proposition is that study of experimental cholesterol-induced atherosclerosis—of the exogenous and endogenous factors controlling it—would yield knowledge of fundamental significance for our understanding of human atherosclerosis.

For many years some investigators rejected these concepts because atherosclerosis had been produced experimentally only in rabbits. The consistent production of gross cholesterol-induced atherosclerosis in omnivorous chicks and dogs and other species now compels rejection of this criticism. For many years some investigators maintained that experimental and clinical atherosclerosis were fundamentally different, since hypercholesteremia was a prerequisite for the former, whereas the latter occurred in many normocholesteremic persons. The consistent production of gross cholesterol-induced atherosclerosis in chicks and rabbits with minimal hypercholesteremia, as well as the demonstration of a "xanthomatous tendency" in many persons with atherosclerosis, now compels rejection of this criticism. During the last decade, particularly, research in both clinical and experimental atherosclerosis has brought overwhelming support to the basic tenet of the cholesterol concept of atherosclerosis. What conclusion must be drawn from this? Certainly present knowledge does not permit us to state that the atherosclerosis problem is solved. Certainly much basic clinical and laboratory research on both exogenous and endogenous aspects of the role of cholesterol in atherosclerosis lies ahead of us before solution is reached. What present knowledge affords us is a fundamental approach for future research—the approach embodied in what we have termed the cholesterol concept of atherogenesis. In this direction, we predict, lies the solution of the atherosclerosis problem, and with it the eventual control and elimination of this malevolent disease.

Acknowledgments

This report is based on the work of a large team which over the last 10 years has included Doctors L. C. Akman, S. A. Carlen, D. V. Dauber, M. Feldman, Jr., G. Gros, R. Harris, L. Horlick, M. Hurwitz, M. Lowenthal, R. S. Megibow, A. J. Miller, R. Pick, S. Rodbard, A. Sanders, J. G. Schlichter, E. N. Silber and J. Stamler and the following technicians: L. Adams, E. Arnold, C. Bolene, G. Crowley, M. Dudley, W. Foote, L. Friedberg, L. Havel, P. Johnson, E. Levinson and J. Meyer.

I am deeply appreciative of the valuable aid of Dr. Stamler in preparing this review.

This work is from the Medical Research Institute, Michael Reese Hospital, Chicago, Ill. Grants-in-aid from the Life Insurance Medical Research Fund and National Heart Institute of the United States Public Health Service constituted the principal sources of support for these studies. Additional funds were obtained from the Special Cardiac Fund of the Committee on Scientific Research, American Medical Association; the Chicago Heart Association; the Sam and Sarah Ehrlich Fund; the A. B. Kuppenheimer Fund; the E. J. Loewenthal Fund; the Herbert G. Mayer Fund; the Michael Reese Research Foundation; the Nelson Morris Fund; the Jeannette N. and Alex D. Nast Fund for Cardiovascular Research; the Emil and Fanny Wedeles Fund.

Bibliography

The reader is referred to the forthcoming review from the department for a complete bibliography: Katz, L. N., and Stamler, J.: Experimental Atherosclerosis. Springfield, Charles C Thomas. In press.

Human Atherosclerosis and the Diet

By ANCEL KEYS, PH.D.

DISCUSSIONS about the possible effects of the diet on the development of human atherosclerosis center on five items: (1) calorie excess and the resulting obesity, (2) cholesterol in the diet, (3) animal fats in the diet, (4) total fats in the diet, (5) the dietary supply of substances which may have a "lipotropic" action, for example, lecithin, choline, inositol. Since the data on the possible action in man of the lipotropic substances pertain to pharmacologic rather than dietary levels and, moreover, are either questionable or negative in regard to an effect on atherosclerosis, the present discussion will not make further mention of these substances.

There are abundant actuarial data which show there is an elevated incidence of fatal atherosclerosis in obese or overweight people. Routine necropsy studies indicate a direct relationship between atherosclerotic changes in the arteries, including the deposition of cholesterol and lipids, and relative fatness of the whole body. Experiments on the production of atherosclerosis in animals likewise show that the relative calorie intake is important.[3] But atherosclerosis occurs in many persons who are neither fat nor overweight. Our first real conclusion, then, is that the development of the atherosclerotic process is abetted, at least in some persons, by an excessive calorie intake and/or the resulting obesity. The calorie level of the diet is an influential but not a controlling factor.

At present the greatest concern about the diet in regard to atherosclerosis has to do with the consumption of foods which contain cholesterol. In some animals, notably the rabbit and the chicken, the addition of large amounts of cholesterol to the diet can lead to high serum cholesterol concentrations and to arterial lesions which resemble human atherosclerosis in many respects.

Unfortunately, these animal experiments do not necessarily have any relevance to the question of the role of the diet in human atherosclerosis. No animal species close to man in metabolic habitus has been shown to be susceptible to the induction of atherosclerosis by cholesterol feeding. The nearest approach to metabolic comparability is the dog which requires extensive thyroid damage as well as tremendous amounts of dietary cholesterol before positive effects can be elicited.

Moreover, even in the favorite species for such experimentation, the herbivorous rabbit, the necessary concentration of cholesterol in the diet is fantastically high in comparison with actual human diets. The actual range of daily intakes of cholesterol provided by real human diets is from zero to perhaps 1000 mg., but the vast majority of human diets seldom average as much as 700 mg. The cholesterol levels in the diets used to induce atherosclerosis in animals range from 0.5 to 5 per cent by weight of the dry food, the most popular level being 2 per cent. This means something like 1000 to 10,000 mg. of cholesterol per 1000 Calories of food, the 2 per cent cholesterol level being equivalent to about 4000 mg. per 1000 Calories if 30 per cent of the calories are derived from fats. We should have to provide some 10,000 to 15,000 mg. of cholesterol daily to a man to be comparable. Moreover, there is reason to believe that man has a greater power of cholesterol regulation than does the rabbit or the chicken. From the animal experiments alone the most reasonable conclusion would be that the cholesterol content of human diets is unimportant in human atherosclerosis.

Direct evidence on man in this connection is unimpressive. Arguments about the incidence of atherosclerosis and the customary intake of cholesterol in the Far East are based on no real data on either atherosclerosis incidence or the character of the diet. The recent analysis of mortality data in Scandinavia[10] is more acceptable but still suffers from the inherent weakness of attempting to discover causation from a parallelism between crude estimates of national averages for two variables. Besides the dubious point of attributing war-time changes in vital statistics to actual changes in atherosclerosis, the analysis glosses over the fact that the presumed variations in cholesterol intake were parallel to similar variations in total dietary fat and, at least to some extent, to changes in calorie intake and physical activity (see also[13]).

Such, in substance, is the actual evidence on human atherosclerosis itself. But significant inferences can be made from indirect evidence if we admit that there is an important relationship between atherosclerosis and the concentration of cholesterol in the serum. There is overwhelming evidence for such a relationship:

(1) On the average, wherever the serum cholesterol tends to be high—as in diabetes, nephrosis, hypothyroidism, and idiopathic hy-

percholesterolemia—there is a tendency toward early and severe atherosclerosis.

(2) Persons with definite evidence for disease of the coronary arteries tend to have elevated serum cholesterol values[4] especially when they are compared with properly matched "normals."[5] Good confirmation can be obtained from recent raw data.[6, figs. 14, 15]

(3) There is at least some parallelism between the age trend of cholesterol concentration in the serum and the age trend in atherosclerosis development.[7, 9]

(4) In animal experiments there is a close parallelism between the serum cholesterol level and the development of experimental "atherosclerosis."

There is much new ev'dence on the effect of the diet on the serum cholesterol level in man. In the first place, the serum cholesterol level of man is independent of large differences in the habitual voluntary intake of cholesterol.[7, 8] Several important confirmations of this fact have been published recently.[4, 14] Colossal intakes, however, far beyond those possible in natural diet, may cause a slow rise in the serum cholesterol.[12]

The rice-fruit diet, which is devoid of both fats and cholesterol, produces a prompt fall in the serum of men with normal levels of cholesterol[2] and a dramatic fall in patients with severe idiopathic hypercholesteremia.[8] We have found that the addition of vegetable fat to this cholesterol-free diet is followed by an equally dramatic rise of serum cholesterol to previous levels.

We have been able recently to make systematic studies on these questions with men under full supervision on diets rigidly controlled for some four months. Starting (and ending) with standard diets providing daily intakes of 150 Gm. of fat and 600 to 700 mg. of cholesterol, the following findings emerged:

(1) Change to a diet devoid of cholesterol and providing 15 Gm. of fat daily produced a rapid fall in serum cholesterol to about 80 per cent of the control value.

(2) Almost identical results were obtained with the same diet to which had been added about 500 mg. of cholesterol daily.

(3) Change to a diet devoid of cholesterol but providing about 70 Gm. of fat daily, produced a decline in serum cholesterol about half as great as when the fat level was only 15 Gm. (No. 1, above).

(4) The addition of 500 mg. of cholesterol daily to the diet (No. 3, above) providing 70 Gm. of fat did not change the result.

It should be noted that all of these experimental diets were comparable in calories and proteins, that the differences in fat intake were achieved by changing the amount of vegetable fat in the diet, and that the differences in cholesterol intake were achieved by adding or withholding whole egg yolks (from which cholesterol is readily absorbed). Finally, with each of the diets the major change in serum cholesterol occurred in the first week or so, and there was a tendency to reach a plateau, or at least a much slower rate of change, in subsequent weeks.

Much longer-term experiments on man are desirable but, so far as they go, these data are consistent within themselves and with all other facts known to me. The ensemble points strongly to the conclusion that, other things being equal, the serum cholesterol level in adult man is independent of the cholesterol intake over the range of zero to at least 700 mg. daily. But the fat intake is quite another matter and appears to have great importance. However, there is not the slightest evidence for a difference between animal and vegetable fat in this regard.[1]

It is now well recognized, and should have been clear long ago, that all animals, including man, have a large capacity for synthesizing cholesterol. Our experiments on fat-free diets also show that man has a large capacity to remove the cholesterol already present in the blood serum. On such diets the rate of removal of cholesterol from the serum seems to be proportional to the initial (control) serum level of cholesterol. In one patient with hypercholesteremia (900 mg. per 100 ml. of serum), the rate of disappearance from the blood was about 1500 mg. daily for several weeks on a fat-free diet. But with the same cholesterol-free diet to which were added about 50 gm. of vegetable fat, there was an increase of cholesterol in his total serum amounting to about 1000 mg. a day for a period of several weeks.

Now, clearly the cholesterol level is not the whole story in the development of atherosclerosis; otherwise the patient mentioned above would have been dead long ago. But, in so far as there is an important relationship between serum cholesterol and atherosclerosis, these dietary data have both theoretic and practical implications of some consequence.

A final question may be raised about the significance of all this in view of the studies by Gofman and his colleagues on the materials separated in the ultracentrifuge. From the evidence reported so far we may make two comments and draw a tentative conclusion:

(1) The response to diet of the serum concentration of substances characterized by -10 to -20 Svedberg units of sedimentation (the "G" substances) appears to be similar to our findings with serum cholesterol, and

(2) There is as yet no reason to suggest that the concentration of G substances in the serum is any more closely related to atherosclerosis than is the concentration of total cholesterol.

(3) At present, we may conclude that the implications for atherosclerosis drawn from dietary effects on serum cholesterol would be similar if the serum criterion were the concentration of the G substances.

In summary, then, we may remark that direct evidence on the effect of the diet on human atherosclerosis is very little and is likely to remain unsatisfactory for a long time. But such evidence as there is, plus valid inferences from indirect evidence, suggests that a substantial measure of control of the development of atherosclerosis in many may be achieved by control of the intake of calories and of all kinds of fats, with no special attention to the cholesterol intake. This means: (1) avoidance of obesity, with restriction of the body weight to about that considered standard for height at age 25; (2) avoidance of periodic gorging and even temporary large calorie excesses; (3) restriction of all fats to the point where the total extractable fats in the diet are not over about 25 to 30 per cent of the total calories; (4) disregard of cholesterol intake except, possibly, for a restriction to an intake less than 1 Gm. per week.

Acknowledgments

This work is from the Laboratory of Physiological Hygiene, University of Minnesota, Minneapolis, Minn.

References

[1] Abelin, I.: Zur Frage der Sterinbildung im Tierkörper. II. Mitteilung. Helvet. physiol. et pharmacol. Acta 6: 879, 1948.

[2] Chapman, C. B., Gibbons, T., and Henschel, A.: The effect of the rice-fruit diet on the composition of the body. New England J. Med. 243: 899, 1950.

[3] FIRSTBROOK, J. B.: Factors influencing the atherosclerotic process. Circulation *2:* 464, 1950.

[4] GEIER, F. M.: Cholesterol and coronary artery disease. Permanente Found. M. Bull. *7:* 49, 1949.

[5] GERTLER, M. M., GARN, S. M., AND WHITE, P. D.: Diet, serum cholesterol and coronary artery disease. Circulation *2:* 696, 1950.

[6] GOFMAN, J. W., JONES, H. B., LINDGREN, F. T., LYON, T. P., ELLIOTT, H. A., AND STRISOWER, B.: Blood lipids and human atherosclerosis. Circulation *2:* 161, 1950.

[7] KEYS, A.: The physiology of the individual as an approach to a more quantitative biology of man. Federation Proc. *8:* 523, 1949.

[8] ——, MICKELSEN, O., MILLER, E. v. O., AND CHAPMAN, C. B.: The relation in man between cholesterol levels in the diet and in the blood. Science *112:* 79, 1950.

[9] ——, ——, ——, HAYES, E. R., AND TODD, R. L.: The concentration of cholesterol in the blood serum of normal man and its relation to age. J. Clin. Investigation *29:* 1347, 1950.

[10] MALMROS, H.: The relation of nutrition to health. A statistical study of the effect of the war-time on arteriosclerosis, cardiosclerosis, tuberculosis and diabetes. Acta med. Scandinav. Suppl. *286:* 137, 1950.

[11] MELLINKOFF, S. M., MACHELLA, T. E., AND REINHOLD, J. G.: The effect of a fat-free diet in causing low serum cholesterol. Am. J. M. Sc. *220:* 203, 1950.

[12] MESSINGER, W. J., POROSOWSKA, Y., AND STEELE, J. M.: Effect of feeding egg yolk and cholesterol on serum cholesterol levels. Arch. Int. Med. *86:* 189, 1950.

[13] SCHETTLER, G.: Zum Einfluss der Ernahrung auf den Cholesteringehalt des Blutes. Klin. Wchnschr. *28:* 569, 1950.

[14] WILKINSON, C. F., JR., BLECHS, E., AND REIMER, A.: Is there a relation between diet and blood cholesterol? Arch. Int. Med. *85:* 389, 1950.

Blood Lipids and Human Atherosclerosis

By John W. Gofman, M.D., Ph.D., Hardin B. Jones, Ph.D., Thomas P. Lyon, M.D., Frank Lindgren, B.S., Beverly Strisower, B.S., David Colman, B.S., and Virgil Herring, B.S.

Previously evidence has been presented relating certain serum lipoproteins to the development of atherosclerosis in man.[1-3] Further studies now enable us to make quantitative estimations of the relationship of certain aspects of lipid transport via lipoproteins with atherosclerogenesis, including follow-up studies. There are several points of evidence which have led us to an understanding of this derangement of blood lipoproteins from the "normal" pattern. The first observation of derangement of the lipid transport mechanism was made on serum lipoproteins of rabbits subsequent to their development of hypercholesteremia by cholesterol feeding.

In the course of cholesterol feeding, molecules of high S_f classes, S_f 10–30, 30–100, and higher (of higher molecular weight, lower density, higher lipid content and lower protein content than the normally occurring lipoproteins) appear in the serum, in contrast to the normal lipoproteins which are in the class of S_f 10 and below. There is differential significance to the presence of these several lipoproteins which appear in the serum under several types of experimental conditions inducing hypercholesteremia. For the rabbit there is no relation between the serum levels of S_f 10 and lower and atherosclerosis[1] during active atherogenesis. A lack of positive relationship between S_f 10 and lower molecules and atherosclerosis has been significantly demonstrated ($r \cong -0.32$).

Some of these observations were on rabbits which received potassium iodide in addition to cholesterol feeding. Under this condition the increase in serum cholesterol and serum lipids is primarily in the S_f 10 and lower fraction, which is elevated as high as or higher than in the cholesterol-fed rabbit that develops atherosclerosis. In fact, severe atherosclerosis often develops with low levels of this class of lipoproteins, whereas no atherosclerosis develops in spite of several fold increase in concentration of such lipoproteins. However, there is a high relationship (correlation coefficient $\cong +0.8$) between estimated degree of atherosclerosis as measured at autopsy and the concentration of lipoproteins of the S_f 10–30 class when it develops *regardless* of the experimental condition. This observation is drawn from rabbits which were rendered hypercholesteremic by: (a) cholesterol feeding, (b) cholesterol and oil feeding, (c) cholesterol and potassium iodide feeding, and (d) cholesterol and oil feeding in the alloxanized rabbit. (Each of these experimental types has a differential alteration of the serum lipoproteins.) Under certain uniform conditions such as cholesterol or cholesterol and oil feeding there is an excellent quantitative relationship between degree of atherosclerosis and the total blood cholesterol. However, this is only due to the fact that the S_f 10–30 molecules account in this case for the main proportion of the increase in total serum cholesterol. That the total blood cholesterol itself is not the important feature has been clearly demonstrated by Pierce[4] in our laboratory, studying the Duff[5] type of alloxanized rabbit. Duff has previously shown that feeding cholesterol to alloxan diabetic rabbits results in elevation of serum cholesterol to levels over 2000 mg. per 100 cc. with a much less severe atherosclerosis developing than in the normal cholesterol-fed rabbit at comparable and much lower total cholesterol levels. Pierce has shown that in the Duff type rabbit the cholesterol is transported primarily in the form of molecules of the S_f 100 and higher classes. Some of the Duff type rabbits develop atherosclerosis, but they are the ones which also develop large amounts of S_f 10–30 molecules as well as the S_f 30 and higher molecules. Recently Graham and co-workers[6] in this laboratory maintained cholesterol- and oil-fed rabbits on daily injections of heparin (10 mg. per kilogram per day). Heparin minimizes a rise in the concentration in the S_f 10–30 class of molecules by facilitating the formation of lower S_f classes of lipoproteins. These rabbits are markedly protected from atherosclerosis even though they are exposed to a metabolic burden of fat (3 Gm. per day) and cholesterol (1 Gm. per day) which ordinarily produces atherosclerosis.

It appears therefore that high levels of S_f 10–30 lipoproteins are consistently associated with atherosclerosis in the rabbit, whereas no association can be established for the S_f 100 and higher and the S_f 10 and lower classes. Serum cholesterol can be used as a partial guide *only* under the special conditions where the S_f 10–30 molecules are relatively greatly increased. If cholesteremia in the Duff-alloxan type rabbit and the Anitschkow-cholesterol-fed rabbit is compared with atherosclerosis, a significant negative relationship will actually be found between atherosclerosis and serum cholesterol. As will be discussed later, each of the different types of rabbit hypercholesteremia, (1) the Duff-alloxan type with its increment of increased cholesterol primarily in the lipoproteins greater than S_f 100; (2) the Anitschkow-cholesterol-fed type with its increase first in the S_f 10 and lower; and (3) the later stage of cholesterol or cholesterol and oil feeding (with the bulk of cholesterol carried in the S_f 10–30 class of lipoproteins), has its counterpart in types of human sera which are probably of similar differential significance (see fig. 1).

Preliminary studies (with the cooperation of Kendall[7] and Chaikoff[8]) on hypercholesteremic-atherosclerotic dogs and chickens indicate that there is a similar shift in both species of the serum lipids to higher S_f lipoproteins than exist normally. It must still be determined, through a more extensive study, which special class may be involved in these species, although it is known that the S_f 10–30 class becomes elevated in both dog and chicken.

A detailed account of the chemical composition and physical nature of the lipoproteins composing the lipid transport system has appeared.[3, 9, 10] Each of the lipoproteins (at least nine discrete components up to S_f 17 and a host of unresolved components above S_f 20 have been observed) contains cholesterol, phospholipid and protein, but in different amounts. Those lipoproteins above S_f 13 contain neutral fat also. Since each lipoprotein can vary in concentration in a semi-independent way, there is no assured relationship between total serum cholesterol or phospholipid or fat and the concentration of any particular lipoprotein species. We have seen no higher correlation than $r \cong 0.4$ to 0.5 between serum cholesterol and any one of these lipoprotein components or between the individual lipoprotein classes. It is the purpose of this paper to evaluate quantitatively the relationship that does exist between total serum cholesterol and the certain classes of lipoproteins in the human and the relation of each to atherosclerosis. We have previously indicated that elevation of the S_f 12–20 lipoproteins,[3, 11] is part of a lipid metabolic defect which is often associated with elevations in level of the S_f 20–100 class of lipoproteins. Further, there are many individuals who have inordinately high S_f 20–100 levels at a modest S_f 12–20 level. (See later section concerning S_f 12–20 intercorrelation with lipoproteins above

S_f 20.) In humans with less severe degrees of the metabolic error, S_f 20–100 levels fluctuate acutely with reference to ingestion of fat. However, in those with severe degrees of the metabolic error the S_f 20–100 class is elevated even postabsorptively.[11] Until now we have refrained from using the lipoproteins higher than S_f 20 as a correlative guide because of the greater fluctuations in concentrations of these lipoproteins than occurs in the S_f 12–20 class. In spite of the variability in levels of molecules from S_f 20–100, it has now become evident, as will be explained below, that these molecules are strongly related to atherosclerosis and represent an independent contribution to accountability for atherosclerosis, in addition to the already established association of the S_f 12–20 class of lipoproteins with atherosclerosis. It should be pointed out that the intercorrelation between the S_f 12–20 and the S_f 20–100 classes of lipoproteins is relatively low, and it is common to see severe disproportion in the concentration of S_f 12–20 and S_f 20–100 classes. Atherosclerosis is associated with elevated levels of either class of lipoproteins, and since the intercorrelation of the two classes is low, a significant improvement in identification of atherosclerogenic states results from consideration of the entire S_f 12–100 class of lipoproteins (that is, the sum S_f 12–20 and S_f 20–100).

The entire S_f 12–100 class of lipoproteins represents only about 10 to 15 per cent of all the serum lipoproteins and contains approximately 10 to 15 per cent of the total serum cholesterol. As will be shown in analysis of the data below, it is the cholesterol within the S_f 12–100 lipoproteins that represents the entirety of the association of cholesterol with atherosclerosis. Since this amount is such a small fraction of the total cholesterol, and is so poorly related to the remaining 85 to 90 per cent of the cholesterol, it is largely masked in the routine determination of total serum cholesterol, even if the latter measurement is done with great accuracy.

In this report we have studied two groups: (1) patients with coronary artery disease manifested by either myocardial infarction or classic angina pectoris, and (2) individuals who are presumably normal in that they show no clinical sign of atherosclerosis and are in active physical condition normal to their mode of living. While other diseases with atherosclerotic complications are discussed, particular use is made of coronary artery disease, for it can be diagnosed with a high degree of reliability. This criterion group is manifesting a complication of atherosclerosis of the coronary arteries in an estimated 90 to 95 per cent of cases.[2] Among normal persons, atherosclerosis is consistently reported with high occurrence rate from autopsy reports.[12] Presumably, for many years of evolution of the atherosclerotic state, there was no external sign of the disease. It is estimated that in any group of supposedly normal, adult men, 30 to 50 per cent may be actively developing arterial atheroma.[11] Statistical comparisons made between presumed normals and atherosclerotics are, in their crude form, of limited quantitative interpretation, since they contrast a population about 95 per cent atherosclerotic to a population 50 to 80 per cent "true normal" admixed with 50 to 30 per cent atherosclerogenic normal. However, it is possible to estimate a correction for the impurity of the latter criterion group, as will be described in a later section.

We have studied 253 normal men and 93 men with coronary artery disease, all between the ages of 41 and 50 years. Of the coronary group, 75 were men studied at least six weeks after a myocardial infarction and 18 were men manifesting typical angina pectoris. In another group of men between the ages of 51 and 60 years, 149 were normal and 126 had coronary disease; in this coronary group there were 110 survivors of myocardial infarction and 16 patients with typical angina pectoris. There were no significant differences in lipoprotein or cholesterol levels between the cases with angina and those with myocardial infarction, so in each age group both types were combined as "patients with coronary artery disease" for purposes of analysis.

Several approaches were made to the analysis of the data in an effort to assess the relationship of S_f 12–20 and S_f 20–100 lipoproteins and of total serum cholesterol to atherosclerosis. Over-all relationships and the relationship of each measure independent of the others were evaluated previously[11]; it was demonstrated that the S_f 12–20 lipoprotein levels were consistently two to four times as effective as the serum cholesterol level in segregating atherosclerotics from normals. It became apparent in those data that there was a slight residual association of serum cholesterol levels with atherosclerosis in the 41 to 50 year age group, even when the relationship of S_f 12–20 lipoprotein levels with atherosclerosis was taken into account. This suggested the probable existence of certain additional lipoprotein classes inde-

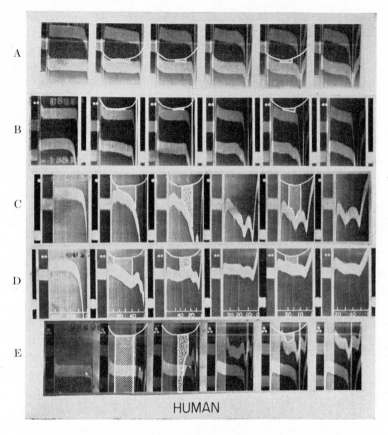

HUMAN

Fig. 1.

Fig. 1. Ultracentrifugal flotation patterns, showing the increase in the lipid metabolic defect in the human and the experimental rabbit. In all these figures the S_f rates can be read off the S_f scale placed on all frames; concentrations of various lipoprotein fractions are proportional to the shaded areas. A shows the flotation pattern of a normal child and a normal rabbit, both having low concentrations of lipoproteins below S_f 10 and trivial concentrations above S_f 10. B shows the patterns for a normal human and for a rabbit with elevation of the concentrations of lipoproteins below S_f 10 but without appreciable elevations of lipoproteins of higher S_f classes. C shows corresponding patterns for human and rabbit with moderate concentrations of lipoproteins of S_f 10 and

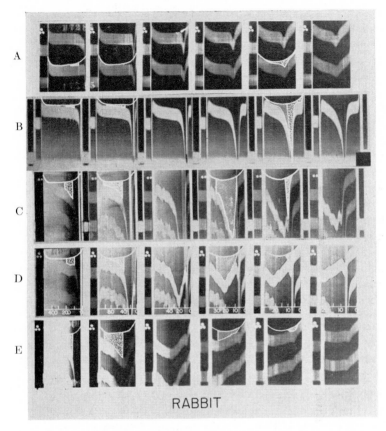

FIG. 1.—Cont'd

less, but with great elevations in the S_f 12–20 and 20–40 classes in the human and S_f 10–30 class in the rabbit. This rabbit developed marked atherosclerosis. D shows analogous patterns for human and rabbit with marked elevation of S_f 12–20 class in human and S_f 10–30 class in rabbit, but with depression of the concentration of lipoproteins of S_f 10 and less. This rabbit also developed marked atherosclerosis. E shows the manifestation of severe lipid metabolic error in human and rabbit. Note the low concentration of lipoproteins below S_f 10, moderate concentration of lipoproteins of S_f 12–20 class in the human and S_f 10–30 class in the rabbit, and high concentration of lipoproteins from S_f 20–100 in both human and rabbit.

pendently associated with atherosclerosis. The current analysis confirms the association of certain lipoproteins (the S_f 12–20 and S_f 20–100 classes) with atherosclerosis and the exclusion of other lipoproteins from such association. The analysis shows further that the total serum cholesterol level is associated with atherosclerosis only through its weak relationship with the important S_f 12–20 and S_f 20–100 classes of lipoproteins. When individuals are evaluated at the same combined level of lipoproteins of the S_f 12–100 class (S_f 12–20 plus S_f 20–100), there is *no* residual relationship of the remaining bulk ($\sim$ 85 to 90 per cent) of the serum cholesterol with atherosclerosis, even in individuals with marked hypercholesteremia. Serum cholesterol measurements permit only a slight segregation of atherosclerotics from normals in the age group under 50 years, and permit no segregation of the atherosclerotic group from the normal group above the age of 50 years. Overall, a serum cholesterol determination tends more to obscure than to clarify the status of an individual with respect to atherosclerosis. By contrast, the S_f 12–100 lipoprotein determination offers a continuous scale of positive association with atherosclerotic activity, no matter whether the serum cholesterol is low, moderate, or high.

Analysis of the Relationship of S_f 12–20 and S_f 20–100 Lipoproteins and of Serum Cholesterol to Atherosclerosis

The literature concerning serum lipids is marked by great differences which are the result both of nonuniformity of populations sampled and of technical differences in laboratory procedures of analysis. It is ridiculous to contrast serum lipid analyses between groups without rigorous control of both of these sources of variation in reported lipid concentration. For this study it has been an absolute requirement to determine both lipoproteins and total serum cholesterol on the same serum sample under controlled laboratory conditions. This approach permits a direct comparison between these two types of lipid analysis as to their association with atherosclerotic tendency.

Table 1 provides a summary of the pertinent data for the various lipoprotein classes measured and for the total serum cholesterols in the 41 to 50 and 51 to 60 year age groups considered. These data are requisite to a further evaluation of the association of any of the measures with atherosclerosis. It is evident that for the 41 to 50 year

age group, all three measures, the S_f 12–20 level, the S_f 35–100*
level, and the total serum cholesterol level, are significantly higher in
patients with coronary artery disease than in normal persons. The first
crude assessment of the association of each measure with atherosclerosis can be made by comparing the difference in mean levels
(between the normal and coronary group) with reference to the stand-

TABLE 1.—*Lipoprotein and Cholesterol Measurements in Normal Subjects and
Patients with Coronary Artery Disease*

	41-50 Year Age Group (Males)		51-60 Year Age Groups (Males)	
	Normal Subjects	Coronary Disease Patients	Normal Subjects	Coronary Disease Patients
No. Cases..................	253	93	149	126
Mean S_f 12–20 Lipoprotein Level....................	45 ± 27	71 ± 32	46 ± 21	70 ± 31
Mean S_f 35–100 Lipoprotein Level....................	64 ± 49	120 ± 74	61 ± 45	92 ± 65
Mean Combined S_f 12–20 + S_f 35–100 Lipoprotein Level	109 ± 65	191 ± 93	107 ± 57	162 ± 79
Mean Serum Cholesterol Level	260 ± 53	297 ± 68	274 ± 65	286 ± 69
Intercorrelations*............				
S_f 12–20 vs. Chol..........	0.40	0.39	0.23	0.25
S_f 35–100 vs. Chol.........	0.3	0.13	0.0	0.0
S_f 12–20 vs. S_f 35–100......	0.41	0.54	0.44	0.38

All values are given plus or minus the standard deviation of the distribution.
* Coefficients of correlation are expressed as Pearson r.

ard deviation of the distribution of values for each measure. Thus it is
seen that the greatest relative difference established for normal subjects and coronary patients 41 to 50 years old is in the combined S_f
12–20 and S_f 35–100 lipoprotein measure. Next is the separation
achieved by the S_f 35–100 lipoprotein measure. An almost equivalent
separation exists for the S_f 12–20 lipoprotein measure. The poorest
separation exists for the serum cholesterol measure. The actual values
of the quotient of difference in means by the σ for each measure is
given in table 2.

* S_f 20–100 class equals S_f 20–35 plus S_f 35–100. As discussed in the text, the
independent contribution of S_f 20–35 is small; it is omitted from this analysis.

Consideration of the ratios in table 2 reveals that for the 41 to 50 year age group measurement of either S_f 12–20 or S_f 35–100 lipoprotein segregates patients with coronary disease from normal subjects with high efficiency. The best segregation of coronary disease patients from normal subjects is achieved by combining the S_f 12–20 and S_f 35–100 lipoprotein values. Since the contribution of the S_f 12–20 and S_f 35–100 measures are in large part independent of each other, it is understandable that the combination is superior to either

TABLE 2.—*Crude Segregation of Patients with Coronary Disease and Normals by the Lipoprotein and Cholesterol Measures*

	Difference in Means (Coronary Disease—Normals)	Standard Deviation of Normal Distribution	Ratio, Difference in Means: Standard Deviation
41–50 Years			
	mg. per 100 cc.	*mg. per 100 cc.*	
Combined S_f 12–20 + S_f 35–100	82	65	1.3
S_f 35–100	56	49	1.1
S_f 12–20	25	27	0.9
Serum Cholesterol	37	53	0.7
51–60 Years			
Combined S_f 12–20 + S_f 35–100	55	57	1.0
S_f 35–100	31	45	0.7
S_f 12–20	24	21	1.1
Serum Cholesterol	12	65	0.19

alone. Individually and combined the lipoprotein measurements are highly superior to serum cholesterol measurement in segregating coronary disease patients from normals. In fact, in the 51 to 60 year age group the serum cholesterol measurement cannot be shown to produce any significant segregation of the coronary disease group from the normal group.

A simple method of measuring the association of each factor (that is, S_f 12–20 level, S_f 35–100 level, or serum cholesterol level) independently with atherosclerosis is achieved by comparing the lipoprotein segregating ability at any particular serum cholesterol level, and conversely the serum cholesterol segregating ability at any particular lipoprotein level. Thus, there are given in figure 2 A, B, C the average values of S_f 12–20 and S_f 35–100 lipoprotein levels for every part of the serum cholesterol range, for both normals and patients with coronary artery disease. It is evident that the patients with coronary artery disease show essentially the same elevation of S_f 12–20 and S_f 35–100 lipoproteins above normal levels when compared *at the same cholesterol level* throughout the entire cholesterol range. This is equivalent to matching each patient with coronary disease with a normal who has the same cholesterol level. Conversely, the data of figure 2C can be used to compare the serum cholesterol level in patients with coronary disease with the level in normal persons at the same lipoprotein level. It is seen that when individuals in the coronary group are matched with normals having the same lipoprotein levels there is no significant difference in cholesterol level, indicating that cholesterol level of itself does *not* segregate coronary and normal populations independently of its weak association with the lipoprotein classes (S_f 12–20 and S_f 35–100) which are truly associated with atherosclerosis. For the two age groups studied, the actual data obtained in such comparisons are given below.

Comparison of S_f 12–20 and S_f 35–100 Lipoproteins in Coronary Disease Patients and in Normal Subjects at Identical Cholesterol Levels

From the data shown in figure 2 A, B, C it can be seen that 41 to 50 year old patients with coronary disease average higher than normal in (S_f 12–20 plus S_f 35–100) lipoproteins by 69 mg. per 100 cc., higher in S_f 35–100 lipoproteins by 51 mg. per 100 cc., higher in S_f 12–20 lipoproteins by 18.0 mg. per 100 cc.; all comparisons are with normal subjects at equal cholesterol levels. Patients 51 to 60 years old with coronary artery disease also show equivalent elevations, namely 22 mg. per 100 cc. higher in S_f 12–20 lipoproteins than equivalent normals for the same cholesterol level.

Comparison of Cholesterol Levels at Corresponding Serum Lipoprotein Concentrations

In the 41 to 50 year old group of patients with coronary artery disease, cholesterol is only 17 mg. per 100 cc. higher than in normals compared at the same S_f 12–20 level. This small residual elevation is

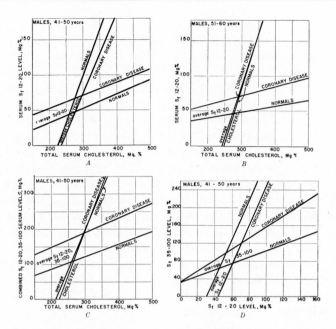

FIG. 2*A*, *B*, *C*. In each diagram separate lines indicate the normal subjects and the coronary disease patients. The lines marked "average cholesterol" indicate the value of the serum cholesterol for a sample of the population chosen at a precise lipoprotein level (either S_f 12–20 or the sum of S_f 12–20 and S_f 35–100, depending upon which plot is considered). The lines marked "average S_f 12–20" indicate the value of the lipoprotein level for a sample of the population chosen at a precise cholesterol level.

These plots show explicitly that the S_f 12–20 or S_f 12–20 plus S_f 35–100 lipoproteins can consistently separate the coronary disease population from the normal population, regardless of the cholesterol level encountered. Shown equally well is the failure of the serum cholesterol level to separate consistently the coronary disease population from the normal population, when these populations are compared at a given lipoprotein level.

D. These plots show the equivalent and independent segregating ability of both the S_f 12–20 and the S_f 35–100 lipoprotein levels for coronary and normal populations.

In all plots the intersection of the two normal curves, or of the two coronary disease curves, gives the mean values for the population concerned; for example, in 2*A*, the mean serum cholesterol and mean S_f 12–20 levels.

completely lost when coronary and normal populations are contrasted at the same (S_f 12–20 plus S_f 35–100) levels; the coronary population is 1 mg. per 100 cc. of cholesterol lower than normals of the same (S_f 12–29 plus S_f 35–109) levels.

In the 51 to 60 year old group, patients with coronary artery disease are likewise unsegregated from normal subjects by cholesterol when cholesterol levels are compared at the same S_f 12–20 level.

Thus it is apparent that lipoproteins of the S_f 12–100 class are highly associated with the atherosclerotic state and that total serum cholesterol is only related to the extent that the small fraction of cholesterol (contained in these particular lipoproteins) can influence the bulk of total serum cholesterol. Inasmuch as approximately 90 per cent of total serum cholesterol is unassociated with atherosclerosis, gross deception is usually to be expected in attempting to evaluate atherosclerosis from the serum cholesterol level on the individual basis. A patient with high atherosclerotic activity will frequently be completely misdiagnosed because his serum cholesterol is moderate or low; conversely, there are many hypercholesteremic individuals who are falsely evaluated as having high atherosclerotic activity. Both of these errors will in general be avoided if the truly atherosclerogenic lipoproteins are used as a clinical guide, rather than the serum cholesterol level.

Figure 2D shows clearly the independent association of the molecules of the S_f 35–100 lipoproteins with atherosclerosis. Even though the S_f 35–100 lipoprotein level is partly related to the S_f 12–20 level, the S_f 35–100 level is higher in patients with coronary artery disease when both normal and atherosclerotic persons are compared at the same S_f 12–20 level. Conversely, the S_f 12–20 level is associated with atherosclerosis independently of its partial relation to S_f 35–100 levels.

The S_f 20–35 class of lipoproteins is also somewhat independently associated with atherosclerosis; however, it is related to both the S_f 12–20 class and the S_f 35–100 class. Hence very little additional gain in assessing atherosclerotic potentialities can be made by including this fraction. A more extensive analysis of our data will be necessary to establish the most effective means of assigning relative weights to the various lipoproteins within the S_f 12–100 class. For the present, due to the larger fluctuation of the S_f 35–100 class, it is advisable to regard the S_f 12–20 and S_f 35–100 classes separately and combined. This does not imply that the S_f 35–100 is of less significance, but rather that its variability may be obscuring an even stronger relationship.

Hypercholesteremic States and Atherosclerotic Activity

Hypercholesteremia (levels over 300 mg. per 100 cc.) has long been considered to be associated with atherosclerosis. However, there is reason to believe that there are differences in atherosclerotic activity even among the hypercholesteremics. To study this question we have compared all the normal subjects (134 cases) having serum cholesterol levels over 300 mg. per 100 cc. with all the patients with myocardial infarction (90 cases) of corresponding age and sex. A slight adjustment between the two groups, correcting to the same serum cholesterol level, was made using the regression equation. (Actual serum cholesterol mean for coronaries was 355; for normals, 347.) When patients with infarcts are compared with normals, both at the same mean cholesterol level (355 mg. per 100 cc.), the S_f 12–20 level in the myocardial infarct group is 89.5 mg. per 100 cc. while that of the normal group is 64.5 mg. per 100 cc. The difference of 25 mg. per 100 cc. is highly significant ($p < 1$ per cent).

If the data for the normals are corrected by the regression equation so that the S_f 12–20 levels are equal in the myocardial infarct and normal groups, the mean cholesterol is not higher in those with infarcts than in the normals.

Of special interest, because of its exceptionally high atherosclerotic activity, is the group manifesting the syndrome xanthoma tuberosum. These patients are quite uniformly hypercholesteremic, but appear to have manifestations of atherosclerosis in excess of what might be anticipated for their degree of hypercholesteremia. Twelve cases of xanthoma tuberosum were matched with hypercholesteremic normals.

The serum cholesterol of the 12 cases of xanthoma ranged from 275 mg. to 640 mg. per 100 cc., averaging 489 mg. per 100 cc. The S_f 12–20 lipoproteins in these cases ranged from 76 mg. per 100 cc. to 520 mg. per 100 cc., averaging 250 mg. per 100 cc. The closest matched group of hypercholesteremic normals that was possible showed a range of 423 to 492 mg. per 100 cc. serum cholesterol, averaging 447 mg. per 100 cc. The S_f 12–20 lipoproteins ranged from 48 mg. per 100 cc. to 99 mg. per 100 cc., except for one case at 300 mg. per 100 cc., and averaged 85 mg. per 100 cc. A slight correction of the normal group to serum cholesterol level identical with the xanthoma patients was made by use of the regression equation. The equivalent normals at 489 mg. per 100 cc. serum cholesterol would have an S_f 12–20 level of 96 mg. per 100 cc. Thus, the extraordinary atherosclerotic tendency of patients with xanthoma tuberosum is explainable because their level of S_f 12–20 lipoproteins is about two and one-half times higher than even equivalently hypercholesteremic normals.

The Accountability for the Atherosclerotic State from Lipoprotein Measurement

In a previous paper,[11] by the technic of biserial correlation, we have estimated roughly the extent of accountability for the atherosclerotic state that can be drawn from the measurement of these serum lipoproteins. These correlation technics are not being used to establish the independent significance of the lipoproteins in atherosclerosis, but rather in an attempt to assess how closely these lipoproteins account for the totality of factors which lead to atherosclerosis. An estimation has been made of the biserial correlation coefficient for the combined S_f 12–20 and the S_f 35–100 measurement with atherosclerosis for the 41 to 50 year age group reported in this paper. This biserial r is 0.57. Ideally one may square such a correlation coefficient to obtain the fraction of the total variance (which is unity) that has been accounted for directly. In this case the total S_f 12–20 and S_f 35–100 have accounted for about four-tenths of factors associated with atherosclerosis. The serum cholesterol measurement contributes nothing further to this estimate. There are limitations to the general use of the biserial technic in an absolute sense in situations of this type; these have been discussed fully in an earlier paper.[11] For, whatever quantitative methods are used to establish relationship between these serum lipoproteins and atherosclerosis, certain factors will always preclude complete accountability of the true relationship that exists. Among these factors are the following:

(1) Accumulated Atherosclerosis vs. Atherosclerotic Activity

Measurement of derangement of lipid metabolism by S_f 12–20 lipoprotein molecules is thought to indicate *active* atherosclerogenesis. Is myocardial infarction caused by *active* or *accumulated* atherosclerosis?

If it is primarily a disturbance of accumulated atheroma, then angina or myocardial infarction is not a pure criterion of active atherosclerosis and is of value only through the relationship of degree of atherosclerosis to rate of accumulation of atherosclerosis. This error has not been estimated and cannot be estimated at this time.

(2) The Impurity of the "Normal" Population

The normal population is composed of a group of true normals whose atherosclerotic activity is insufficient to produce significant atherosclerosis, and normals whose atherosclerosis has not yet advanced to clinically detectable levels or to manifest complications of atherosclerosis. It is variously estimated that 30 to 50 per cent of normals are moderately to severely atherosclerotic.[12]

(3) Focal Factors in Atherosclerosis

The focal character of atherosclerosis, especially when of mild degree is indisputable, but this is consistent with the role of lipids in its pathogenesis. It is entirely reasonable that, given the necessary lipid metabolic abnormality, certain susceptible sites will be earlier and more extensively involved. It may well be the case that if such lipid metabolic abnormality is not present, even susceptible focal sites will not show appreciable disease. In this factor alone there can be great individual variation, even though we feel it is justifiable to say that atherosclerosis of the coronary arteries (and its rate of development) will on the average be more pronounced in patients with myocardial infarction than in normals. The exact degree to which this factor prevents accounting for the total variance between atherosclerotic and normal subjects cannot be estimated at this time. This factor is of importance and it is hoped that follow-up autopsy will enable an assessment of its magnitude.

(4) Reliability, Errors and Consistency of Measurements

Any measured relationships between such factors as total serum cholesterol or S_f 12–20 lipoproteins with atherosclerosis are influenced by errors of measurement and biologic variation with time. Such errors and biologic variation have the effect of reducing the measured relationships, as they have been calculated in this discussion from single measurements on all subjects, normal or atherosclerotic. We have previously made an effort to assess these factors in order that the observed S_f 12–20 or cholesterol relationship to atherosclerosis may be corrected for this attenuation.[11]

The over-all reproducibility from determination to determination on the same individual has a coefficient of reliability of 0.67 ± 0.05 for S_f 12–20 determination and 0.75 ± 0.07 for total serum cholesterol determination. (These figures represent the reliabilities over the one-year period during which the data reported in this paper were collected.) During the same interval the technical reproducibility of the two measurements showed coefficients of reliability of 0.80 ± 0.04 for S_f 12–20 measurement and 0.91 ± 0.001 for serum cholesterol measurement. Therefore it is estimated that the biologic variation during this period is expressed by a coefficient of reliability of $r = 0.84 \pm 0.06$ for S_f 12–20 measurement and $r = 0.82 \pm 0.07$ for total serum cholesterol measurement.

This may be translated into terms of observed biologic variation for the average "normal" (41 to 50 years) whose S_f 12–20 level is 45 mg. per 100 cc. From the standard deviation of the distribution of levels ($\sigma = 27$ mg. per 100 cc.) and the reliability coefficient $r = 0.84$, we calculate a standard error of the obtained value of approximately 10 mg. per 100 cc. S_f 12–20 lipoproteins. For serum cholesterol, the average "normal" whose level is 260 mg. per 100 cc., with a standard deviation of the cholesterol distribution of 63 mg. per 100 cc. and $r = 0.82$, will show a standard error of the obtained value of 25 mg. per 100 cc. cholesterol. Thus, a single measurement places the average individual within +10 mg. per 100 cc. S_f 12–20 and ±25 mg. per 100 cc. serum cholesterol of his "true" value for that particular year period two-thirds of the time.

For over-all variation, including biologic variation and technical errors of measurement, a single determination has a standard error of the obtained value of 15 mg. per 100 cc. S_f 12–20 and 29 mg. per 100 cc. serum cholesterol. Thus a single measurement places an individual (including both biologic variation and technical error) within ±15 mg. per 100 cc. S_f 12–20 and ±29 mg. per 100 cc. cholesterol of the "true" values two-thirds of the time.

The crude biserial r found for the S_f 12–20 plus S_f 35–100 lipoproteins gives a correlation with atherosclerosis of approximately ±0.57. When corrected for (1) the fact that the populations of "normals" and coronary disease patients are only impurely identified, and (2) technical errors that separate a single determination of serum lipoproteins from its true value, the true biserial r may be much greater than the 0.57 measured and may be sufficiently close to unity to account for all the etiologic factors in this disease.

Significance of S_f 12–20 Lipoprotein Levels in the Prognosis and Management of Atherosclerosis

In the preceding section quantitative evidence has been presented for the relationship of S_f 12–20 lipoprotein levels to atherosclerotic activity. It follows therefore that the S_f 12–20 levels might be of prognostic value in patients with established atherosclerosis, in assessing their present potential of atheroma production, as well as in normals, in predicting their likelihood of developing a clinical manifestation of atherosclerosis. We have sufficient follow-up data now to evaluate both of these possibilities.

Prediction of Occurrence of Myocardial Infarction in the Normal Population

A follow-up study has been in progress for the past one and one-half years to obtain information on the occurrence of clinical manifestations of atherosclerosis in individuals previously classified as normal and measured for their S_f 12–20 lipoprotein level. At this time we have complete follow-up information from a block of 1500 normal subjects studied. There have been four occurrences of myocardial infarction documented in males previously normal. These occurred at ages 38, 42, 45 and 53 with S_f 12–20 levels of 100, 68, 55, and 52, respectively. At the same ages in the normal group there are 1000 cases, of whom 340 were above 50 mg. per 100 cc. at the time of study and 660 were below 50 mg. per 100 cc. While the number of cases of occurrence of myocardial infarction is small, the chance that the relationship between S_f 12–20 levels greater than 50 mg. per 100 cc. and occurrence of infarction is not significant is only 1 in 50.

In a group of hypertensives (200) that had shown no clinical evidence of atherosclerosis at the time their S_f 12–20 levels were determined, there have now been three occurrences of myocardial infarction at levels of 55, 78, and 145 mg. per 100 cc. These numbers are not significant by themselves, but they further show that the range of 50 mg. per 100 cc. S_f 12–20 and above includes the probable occurrences of myocardial infarction, since 50 mg. per 100 cc. is the 50:50 division of the hypertensive population. There are many uncomplicated hypertensives in the normal S_f 12–20 ranges.

Recurrence of Myocardial Infarction in Patients with Established Coronary Artery Disease

In a group of patients with previously known coronary artery disease, a rate of occurrence of myocardial infarction higher than in a normal population is expected. We have now been able to observe 39 recurrent myocardial infarctions in the over-all coronary disease population (359 cases) for which we have follow-up information over a one year period. Of these recurrences, 36 showed a level of S_f 12–20 lipoproteins at the time of initial study over 50 mg. per 100 cc., and three had levels below 50 mg. per 100 cc. The actual levels in the recurrences were: 210, 156, 136, 136, 125, 116, 114, 114, 109, 101, 100, 97, 92, 88, 88, 88, 88, 85, 84, 84, 84, 83, 78, 78, 76, 76, 65, 65, 64, 62, 62, 61, 54, 52, 51, 50, 44, 43, and 38 mg. per 100 cc. S_f 12–20 lipoproteins.

There are no factors of difference between the over-all nonrecurrence coronary population and the recurrence population, at least with regard to age, physical activity, sex, previous clinical history, or drug therapy. Some of both the recurrence and nonrecurrence group had been on low fat–low cholesterol diets. Since there are no significant differences between the two groups in other respects, it is justifiable to compare them on the basis of their initial S_f 12–20 lipoprotein levels. Considering a level of 50 mg. per 100 cc. S_f 12–20 lipoproteins, 36 of the recurrences were above this level and three were below this level, whereas in the nonrecurrence group 202 were above and 118 were below this level. A test of significance of the relationship of levels above 50 mg. per 100 cc. with recurrence of myocardial infarction indicates there is less than 1 chance in 1000 that this point of segregation is not real. An even more striking difference is seen above 80 mg. per 100 cc. when the recurrence and nonrecurrence groups are contrasted. In the recurrence group 22 cases were above 80 mg. per 100 cc. and 17 cases were below; in the nonrecurrence group, 64 cases were above 80 mg. per 100 cc. and 256 cases were below. A test of the relationship of S_f 12–20 levels above 80 mg. per 100 cc. with recurrence of myocardial infarction indicates there is less than 1 chance in 10,000 that this point of segregation is not real. These results may be converted to another form of some practical predictive value. The data are plotted in figure 3 as the per cent chance of recurrence of myocardial infarction in one year as a function of a single measured level of S_f 12–20 lipoproteins (along with the data for occurrence of myocardial infarction in one year for individuals who have not previously manifested coronary artery disease). The plot indicates that for a patient with coronary artery disease the over-all chance of a recurrence within one year is approximately 17 per cent for an S_f 12–20 level of 100 mg. per 100 cc., whereas it is approximately 6 per cent for an S_f

TABLE 3.—S_f 12–20 Lipoprotein Level in 49 Patients during First Week after Acute Myocardial Infarction

Level of S_f 12-20 Lipoproteins	Cases Studied during Acute Phase	
	Survived	Died of Infarct
Above 95 mg. per 100 cc.	0	6
Above 80 mg. per 100 cc.	0	13
Above 60 mg. per 100 cc.	6	20
Below 60 mg. per 100 cc.	17	6
Total	23	26

12–20 level of 50 mg. per 100 cc. These data show that the prognosis for a patient with coronary artery disease is much worse if the S_f 12–20 lipoprotein level is high than if it is moderate or low.

A study of 49 patients in the acute phase of myocardial infarction shows that the S_f 12–20 lipoprotein level determined during the first week after occurrence (or from autopsy blood for some of the fatal cases) is of prognostic significance here also. The data are presented in table 3.

It is seen that the levels are much higher in those not surviving the episode of myocardial infarction than in those who do survive. A significance test splitting the survivors and nonsurvivors at 80 mg. per 100 cc. gives a probability of 1 in 10,000 that the observed difference is not significant. Since the two groups were comparable in age, sex, and previous history, it is justifiable to regard the only difference as the lipoprotein level difference. It will be noted that among the survivors the average level is lower than for those myocardial infarction survivors studied at least six weeks beyond the acute episode (see fig. 3). We have frequently observed rises in level in a given patient after the acute phase of a myocardial infarct is past. This probably indicates that in infarction survivors there is a lability of lipid metabolism incidental to the acute insult, which in itself may have increased

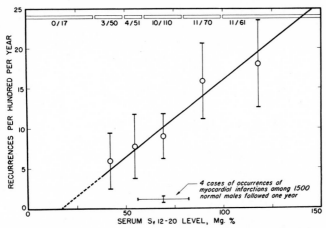

Fig. 3. Shows the per cent chance of recurrence of myocardial infarction in patients with coronary artery disease as a function of S_f 12–20 lipoprotein level. It is based upon 39 recurrent myocardial infarctions in one year follow-up of 359 patients with known coronary artery disease. The class intervals are indicated for each calculation made of the recurrences and the number of patients with myocardial infarction that have been studied. The present best estimate for the position of the similar function for the occurrence of myocardial infarction, de novo, in normals is also shown.

the chance of survival. From studies reported elsewhere,[6] it seems possible that this lipoprotein alteration may be related to increased release of heparin or a heparin-like substance. The higher levels observed in the nonsurvivors suggest the possibility that the more extensive atherosclerogenesis and/or accumulated atheroma most likely present in this group has unfavorably influenced the prognosis.

The data on recurrences of myocardial infarction and the prognosis during the acute phase of an infarct indicate that the over-all outlook for the patient above 80 mg. per 100 cc. S_f 12–20 lipoproteins is quite poor when he develops coronary disease. It is therefore of real importance to evaluate the possibility of giving such patients some protection against their intense atherosclerotic activity, which we have considered possible by means of reducing the S_f 12–20 lipoprotein level via a reduction of the burden of dietary fat.

Our previous and continuing studies of controlled experimental groups have shown that it is possible in most humans to reduce the S_f 12–20 and the S_f 20–100 classes of lipoproteins by restricting the total dietary fat and cholesterol intake.[2, 3] We are fully cognizant of the evidence that fat and cholesterol are synthesized in the body, but this is in no way inconsistent with the observed fact that a partial reduction in S_f 12–20 and S_f 20–100 lipoprotein levels is achieved by a reduction of total fat intake. The first analysis of a dietary follow-up among patients with coronary artery disease can now be made. Of especial pertinence is a comparison of those patients with high S_f 12–20 lipoprotein levels who have experienced recurrent infarction during the period of follow-up with a group of patients of comparable levels who have not shown recurrence during the one year of follow-up. The only therapeutic measure directed toward reduction of lipoprotein levels was the advice and directions for a low fat-low cholesterol diet. A diet of less than 50 Gm. of fat and 200 mg. of cholesterol per day was advised, but it is evident that one cannot assess how rigorously a given patient adhered to this regimen. Therefore, the objective criterion of serial lipoprotein determination was used solely as the measure of dietary response.

Fifty-six cases of myocardial infarction with very high levels (above 80 mg. per 100 cc. S_f 12–20) followed with serial lipoprotein determinations for one year are considered. Out of this group there were 16 recurrent myocardial infarctions during the one year follow-up. Since the patient's statement as to adherence to a low fat diet is untrustworthy, we have eliminated such information from the analysis. A segregation of this group is presented only on the basis of the reduction or nonreduction of the lipoprotein level for the period of follow-up. In this sample it appears there is a differential favoring *nonrecurrence* of myocardial infarction at any relatively reduced level of S_f 12–20 lipoproteins achieved by diet, but for the purpose of demonstrating a significant effect we have divided the group on the basis of whether the level has been reduced and maintained below 70 mg. per 100 cc. or whether the level has remained above 80 mg. per 100 cc. The following fourfold table (table 4) sharply defines the observed result.

Application of a test of significance has shown a probability of one chance in 100 that this segregation is not significant. Therefore the observation that the recurrences have been in the group that main-

TABLE 4.—*Relation of Recurring Myocardial Infarction and S_f 12–20 Lipoproteins Sustained at or Reduced from High Levels*

	Recurrence Group	Non-recurrence Group	Totals
Cases starting and maintaining average level above 80 mg. per 100 cc. S_f 12–20	17	26	43
Cases starting above 80 mg. per 100 cc. but reducing and maintaining level below 70	0	14	14
Totals	17	40	57

TABLE 5.—*Initial S_f 12–20 Level and Average Level during Period of Follow-up for Two Groups Shown in Table 4*

	Recurrence Group			Nonrecurrence Group		
	Initial Level	Average Level	% Reduction	Initial Level	Average Level	% Reduction
Cases starting and maintaining average level above 80 mg. per 100 cc.	112	105	6	116	99	15
Cases starting above 80 mg. per 100 cc. but reducing and maintaining level below 70	—	—	—	104	57	45

tained a high level is highly significant, and we can conclude that dietary reduction of S_f 12–20 level has given significant protection against recurrence of myocardial infarction during this year period of observation. In table 5 are the initial S_f 12–20 level and the average level for the period of follow-up for each of the groups of table 4.

The various groups turn out to be closely matched for initial S_f 12–20 levels. The only exception is the nonrecurrence group which started above 80 mg. per 100 cc. and reduced to an average level below 70 mg. per 100 cc. Here the slightly lower initial level (by 8 mg. per 100 cc.) is the result of the lack of a single matched case at 200 mg. per 100 cc. in this group, compared with the other two groups. In the light of our recent findings that the S_f 20–100 class of lipoproteins are also highly associated with atherosclerosis, and that they are more easily influenced by the restriction of fat, it is likely that reduction in S_f 20–100 may also have afforded part of the protection observed.

Discussion and Summary

1. A variety of serum lipid disturbances experimentally induced in the rabbit, some of which are associated with the development of atherosclerosis, have been analyzed. The S_f 10–30 class of lipoproteins, which develops in the rabbit in certain of these experimental procedures, is highly associated with and universally concurrent with the development of atherosclerosis, independent of the type of metabolic disturbance experimentally induced. The normally occurring lipoproteins (S_f 10 and less), even when elevated experimentally, show no significant positive association with atherosclerosis. Certain other cholesterol-bearing lipoproteins (S_f 100 and higher) are either not associated with atherosclerosis or are inversely associated with atherosclerosis.

2. In the rabbit, total serum cholesterol levels, considering as a group all the types of induced lipid metabolic disturbances, are either unrelated to atherosclerosis, or may be inversely associated with atherosclerosis. Only under the special condition where the major fraction of the cholesterol is in the S_f 10–30 class of lipoproteins does total serum cholesterol correlate well, positively, with atherosclerosis.

3. An estimate of the quantitative association of the S_f 12–20, S_f 20–35, S_f 35–100 lipoprotein classes and of total serum cholesterol with atherosclerogenesis in the human has been made, studying each on the same serum sample from a given individual. Patients with coronary artery disease have served as a criterion group for the atherosclerotics. Throughout the entire age range evaluated, from 41 to 60 years, the S_f 12–20 lipoprotein levels show at least a twofold, and up to a possibly tenfold, higher relationship with atherosclerosis than does the total serum cholesterol. The S_f 20–100 lipoproteins (containing the S_f 20–35 class plus the S_f 35–100 class) also show a correspond-

ingly higher relationship with atherosclerosis than does the total serum cholesterol. The S_f 12–20 lipoproteins and the S_f 35–100 lipoproteins are partially intercorrelated; but each shows, in addition, strong independent associations with atherosclerosis. The S_f 20–35 lipoproteins show a lesser association with atherosclerosis than either of the other classes, and, further, much of the association that is present depends upon partial correlation of the S_f 20–35 lipoprotein with either S_f 12–20 or S_f 35–100 or with both.

The S_f 12–20 and S_f 35–100 lipoproteins show strong association with atherosclerosis, regardless of age or total serum cholesterol level. Thus, even for individuals with the same total serum cholesterol, be it low, moderate, or high, there is strong ability of the S_f 12–20 and S_f 35–100 lipoproteins to segregate atherosclerotics from normals.

Total serum cholesterol shows a much lower ability to segregate atherosclerotics from normals in the 41 to 50 year age group than the S_f 12–20 and S_f 35–100 lipoproteins. In the age group 51 to 60, while the lipoproteins maintain their strong association with atherosclerosis, there is only a borderline ability, if any, of the serum cholesterol to segregate atherosclerotics from normals.

4. What little association total serum cholesterol does have with atherosclerosis is wholly due to its partial correlation with the S_f 12–20 and S_f 20–100 lipoproteins, which are strongly associated with atherosclerosis. In essence, this means that approximately 10 per cent of the serum cholesterol is important for atherosclerosis (namely, the fraction in the S_f 12–20 and S_f 20–100 lipoproteins), while the remaining bulk, approximately 90 per cent, of the cholesterol is unassociated with atherosclerosis. As a result of the fact that the vast bulk of the serum cholesterol is in nonatherogenic lipoproteins, the measurement of total serum cholesterol in an over-all way, does more to obscure the atherosclerotic potentialities of an individual than to clarify them.

5. Even marked hypercholesteremia is not uniformly associated with atherosclerosis. The groups manifesting advanced atherosclerosis (including patients with coronary disease or xanthoma tuberosum) are strikingly segregated from equivalently hypercholesteremic individuals without manifest atherosclerosis by the S_f 12–20 and S_f 35–100 lipoprotein measurements.

6. The crude estimate of the factors which segregate atherosclerotics from normals, based upon biserial correlation, indicates that the com-

bined S_f 12–20 and S_f 35–100 lipoproteins account for at least 35 per cent of the total etiologic factors. When the impurity of the normal population (i.e., admixture with atherosclerotics), the fallibility of diagnosis in the criterion group with coronary disease, the focal factors in atheroma formation, the difference between accumulated atherosclerosis and atherosclerotic activity, and the biologic and technical variation of measurement are all taken into consideration, the combined S_f 12–20 and S_f 35–100 lipoproteins will account for at least 75 to 80 per cent of the total variation between atherosclerotics and normals, and may very well account for the entire difference.

7. Follow-up studies have shown that early recurrence of myocardial infarction in patients with coronary disease is positively and highly related to the S_f 12–20 lipoprotein levels. The recurrence rate of myocardial infarction is approximately 20 per cent per year for those patients with S_f 12–20 levels of 100 mg. per 100 cc., whereas the recurrence rate is approximately 6 per cent for those patients with S_f 12–20 levels of 50 mg. per 100 cc. It may be that when the combined S_f 12–20 and S_f 35–100 levels are evaluated, the relationship of recurrence with lipoprotein level may become stronger.

8. The occurrence of myocardial infarction, de novo, in normals is positively related to elevation in S_f 12–20 lipoprotein levels.

9. The depression of high S_f 12–20 levels by dietary restriction of fat and cholesterol has been shown to decrease significantly the chance of recurrence of myocardial infarction in patients with established coronary artery disease. At this time a significant statement on the point of dietary protection can be made on a follow-up of high-level patients with coronary disease (above 80 mg. per cent S_f 12–20) only because their recurrence rate has provided significant data in a short period.

10. The demonstration that the S_f 35–100 lipoproteins, in addition to the S_f 12–20 lipoproteins, are associated with atherosclerosis is of especial significance with respect to the ingestion of fat. This class of lipoproteins, the S_f 35–100 class, may be raised acutely in a high proportion of humans following ingestion of fat. In patients with a severe degree of the lipid metabolic derangement which leads to "abnormal" lipoprotein patterns, this S_f 35–100 class of molecules is sustained even postabsorptively. It appears, since we have already demonstrated that a dietary lowering of the S_f 92–29 lipoproteins has

an ameliorative effect on coronary disease (based upon atherosclerosis), that dietary fat restriction is equally important, by way of depressing the S_f 35–100 level, in the effort to control atherosclerosis.

11. The rating of a patient with respect to atherosclerogenic potentialities is best achieved by a measure of the levels of S_f 12–20 lipoprotein and S_f 35–100 lipoproteins. Of the two measures, the S_f 12–20 level is the more stable, not being acutely influenced by diet. The S_f 35–100 level, even though more variable acutely with diet, is nevertheless highly associated with atherosclerosis and provides valuable additional assessment with regard to atherosclerogenesis. Thus we may regard the S_f 12–100 lipoproteins as the "atherosclerogenic band" of the serum lipoproteins. The exact assessment of relative atherogenicity of each subsegment within this region is not now possible, so that, for the present, classification is made without weighting within this region.

Acknowledgments

As part of a long-term evaluation of the prognostic significance of lipoproteins in atherosclerosis, several groups are participating in the provision and evaluation of clinical subjects, in both normal and disease categories. The results of this follow-up will be published jointly by the cooperating groups. Some of the clinical material reported on in this paper has been furnished by such groups, for whose cooperation the authors are grateful. The groups involved are The Framingham Heart Project of the United States Public Health Service (Thomas Dawber, M.D.), The Los Angeles Civil Service Commission (Edward Phillips, M.D.), The Eastman Kodak Corporation (David Fassett, M.D.), The Pan American Airlines (Frederick Leeds, M.D.) The United Airlines (A. C. Ladd, M.D.), the Permanente Hospital (Morris Collen, M.D., and David DeKruif, M.D.), The Fort Miley Veterans Hospital (Gerald Whipple, M.D., and Gordon Hein, M.D.), The Medical Department of San Quentin Prison (Leo Stanley, M.D., and Justin Fuller, M.D.). Individual physicians furnishing material are Hyman Enge'berg, M.D., Francis Chamberlain, M.D., Harry Akesson, M.D., Frank Anker, M.D., Norman Leet, M.D., William Donald, M.D., Alexander Yankley, M.D., Mary Lou Eilert, M.D., Dale Groom, M.D., Henry Kempe, M.D., and John Sampson, M.D.

We wish to acknowledge especially the encouragement and support of Mrs. Albert Lasker.

This work is from the Donner Laboratory of Medical Physics and the Radiation Laboratory, University of California, Berkeley, Calif. It was supported in part by the United States Public Health Service, the Atomic Energy Commission, the General Mills Corporation and the Lederle Laboratories Division of the American Cyanamid Corporation.

REFERENCES

1 GOFMAN, J. W., LINDGREN, F., ELLIOTT, H., MANTZ, W., HEWITT, J., STRISOWER, B., AND HERRING, V.: The role of lipids and lipoproteins in atherosclerosis. Science *3:* 166, 1950.

2 ——, JONES, H. B., LINDGREN, F. T., LYON, T. P., ELLIOTT, A., AND STRISOWER, B.: Blood lipids and human atherosclerosis. Circulation *2:* 161, 1950.

3 ——, LINDGREN, F. T., JONES, H. B., LYON, T. P., AND STRISOWER, B.: Lipoproteins and atherosclerosis. J. Gerontol. *6:* 105, 1951.

4 PIERCE, F.: The serum lipoproteins in the cholesterol fed alloxanized rabbit. Circulation. In press.

5 DUFF, G. L., AND MCMILLAN, G. C.: The effect of alloxan diabetes on experimental cholesterol atherosclerosis in the rabbit. I. The inhibition of experimental cholesterol atherosclerosis in alloxan diabetes. II. The effect of alloxan diabetes on the retrogression of experimental cholesterol atherosclerosis. J. Exper. Med. *89:* 611, 1949.

6 GRAHAM, D. M., LYON, T. P., GOFMAN, J. W., JONES, H. B., YANKLEY, A., AND SIMONTON, J.: Blood lipids and human atherosclerosis. II. The influence of heparin upon lipoprotein metabolism. Circulation *4:* 666, 1951.

7 KENDALL, F., DAVIDSON, J., GOFMAN, J. W., AND JONES, H. B.: Ultracentrifugal studies of the lipoproteins in dogs developing atherosclerosis. To be published.

8 CHAIKOFF, I. L., GOFMAN, J. W., JONES, H. B., AND NICHOLS, N.: Ultracentrifugal studies of the lipoproteins in chicken atherosclerosis induced with stilbestrol. To be published.

9 LINDGREN, F. T., ELLIOTT, H. A., AND GOFMAN, J. W.: The ultracentrifugal characterization and isolation of human blood lipids and lipoproteins, with applications to the study of atherosclerosis. J. Phys. & Colloid Chem. *55:* 80, 1951.

10 LINDGREN, F. T., NICHOLS, A., AND FREEMAN, K.: Chemical characterization of the lipoproteins of human serum. To be published.

11 JONES, H. B., GOFMAN, J. W., LINDGREN, F. T., LYON, T. P., GRAHAM, D. M., STRISOWER, B., AND NICHOLS, A. V.: Lipoproteins in atherosclerosis. Am. J. Med. *11:* 271, 1951.

12 WHITE, N. K., EDWARDS, J. E., AND DRY, T. J.: The relationship of the degree of coronary atherosclerosis with age, in men. Circulation *1:* 645, 1950.

The Management of Acute Cardiac Emergencies

By CLARENCE E. DE LA CHAPELLE, M.D., AND O. ALAN ROSE, M.D.

ALTHOUGH the majority of emergencies of cardiac origin occur in patients with structural heart disease, many involve individuals without demonstrable organic lesions. Those affecting the latter are usually due to changes in rhythm. The most common of these are the paroxysmal supraventricular tachycardias.

Most cardiac emergencies are readily diagnosed by bedside examination, but occasionally, and especially in the presence of arrhythmias, the use of precision records such as the electrocardiogram is necessary to make an accurate diagnosis. It is, of course, essential to interpret correctly the nature of any emergency in order to institute proper treatment. In this article the methods used in recognizing the various emergencies will not be stressed and only the therapeutic procedures employed in their management will be discussed.

Paroxysmal Supraventricular Tachycardias

Auricular Tachycardia

This is the most common of all paroxysmal tachycardias and occurs most often in individuals who are free from structural heart disease. In such patients the paroxysms are usually of short duration and require little or no therapy. Despite the benign nature of these episodes, medical help is not infrequently sought, especially during the initial attacks, or for paroxysms which do not respond to simple measures which most patients learn to use after experiencing repeated attacks. Among the latter are the Valsalva procedure of attempted forced expiration with the glottis shut, prolonged holding of the breath, compression of the neck, and the assumption of various positions, such as lowering the head over the side of a couch, or twisting the head in extreme rotation to either side. Lastly, patients often induce vomiting by mechanical irritation of the pharynx or by drinking mustard diluted in water.

Although death is uncommon in adults during auricular paroxysmal tachycardia, even when organic heart disease is present, serious complications, including heart failure, may occasionally ensue. In infants and young children, however, heart failure and death may occur in the absence of recognizable heart disease. When structural heart disease is present, symptoms including dyspnea, substernal pain, vertigo and syncope may result. Persistence of this rapid arrhythmia may produce heart failure. In such circumstances it is imperative that the impaired heart be spared the excessive burden of the tachycardia by abolishing the abnormal mechanism as soon as possible.

Since most patients with paroxysmal tachycardia suffer from considerable apprehension during an attack, especially during the initial episodes, a sedative in the form of a rapidly acting barbiturate should be administered as promptly as possible. The patient should be placed at rest and reassured of the innocence of the attack. These measures alone will frequently produce reversion to normal rhythm. As a rule morphine and other opiates are contraindicated because of the danger of possible habituation. This is particularly true if the patient does not have underlying heart disease.

If the paroxysm still persists then other methods of therapy should be used. Among these are several physical procedures. Carotid sinus pressure is the one most often tried, and probably the most successful in abolishing paroxysmal tachycardia of auricular and nodal origin. Carotid pressure is most likely to be effective if the sinuses are massaged, trying first the right and then the left. This is best performed by pressing against the carotid sinus at the angle of the jaw, compressing the carotid posteriorly and medially against the vertebral bodies. Considerable pressure in the massaging is required. If this measure is not successful before medication, it is frequently effective in converting supraventricular tachycardias after the patient has been treated with one of the drugs which produce vagal stimulation. The latter include the digitalis substances and Mecholyl. Their uses will be described below. Ocular pressure is also a physical measure to produce vagal stimulation. It is not as effective and apparently is now less often used than carotid sinus massage. Occasionally damage to the eye may result from this treatment.

Although quinidine still seems to be the drug preferred by many clinicians to terminate auricular and nodal paroxysmal tachycardias, one of the rapidly acting glycosides of digitalis is being used more frequently as the drug of choice.[1] In infants and young children who become critically ill in the presence of auricular paroxysmal tachycardias, intravenous administration of a digitalis preparation is not only effective but may actually be life-saving. Digitalis may be given by mouth in the usual digitalizing dosage if there is no urgency.

Ouabain, given intravenously, is probably the best preparation for the rapid conversion of auricular or nodal paroxysmal tachycardia. There is danger in employing this, or any other digitalis preparation, if the patient has received digitalis within the previous two weeks. The initial dose for adults is 0.5 mg. followed every hour by 0.1 mg. until the paroxysm ceases or a total of 1.0 mg. has been administered. Most patients obtain full therapeutic effect with 0.8 mg. of ouabain.

If ouabain is not available, lanatoside C (Cedilanid) may be administered intravenously.[2] The initial dose is 0.8 mg., followed by 0.4 mg. if no favorable response is obtained in one hour. The majority of patients will respond to the initial dose of 0.8 mg. However, a total of 1.6 mg. of lanatoside C may be required. Digoxin,[3] also given intravenously, is another preparation which may be employed for rapid digitalization in the management of auricular and nodal paroxysmal tachycardias. When administered intravenously the introductory dose of 0.5 mg. is followed every two hours by 0.25 mg. until full effect is obtained, or until a total of 1.5 mg. has been given.

Recently another digitalis-like substance, acetyl strophanthidin, has aroused interest but mainly from an experimental standpoint. Apparently this drug, when given intravenously, "causes an almost immediate effect on the ventricular rate of auricular fibrillation."[4] Based on clinical work reported to date, it may prove to be of value in the treatment of acute left ventricular failure, where speed is essential, and in the management of auricular paroxysmal tachycardia. At present, there is not sufficient clinical experience to warrant accurate conclusions as to the indications or value of this drug.

Quinidine, while probably less effective than digitalis, is still preferred by many physicians, at least for preliminary trial, in the treatment of supraventricular tachycardia. When using this drug it is wise to give a test dose of 0.2 Gm. to rule out an idiosyncrasy, although true allergic reactions to quinidine are rarely encountered.[5] After waiting one hour, quinidine sulfate, in doses of 0.4 Gm. to 0.6 Gm., should be given orally every two or three hours for five doses. If the attack has not terminated with this schedule of administration, increased dosages of 0.8 Gm. or 1.0 Gm. may be used in a similar manner for subsequent trials. If conversion has not occurred at these high levels it is best to discontinue quinidine, as success is unlikely. Procaine amide (Pronestyl) may be effective in the conversion of this arrhythmia. The use and dosage of this drug will be discussed below under the treatment of ventricular tachycardia.

Another medication which is effective in the management of this arrhythmia is Mecholyl chloride (acetyl-beta-methylcholine chloride). It is given subcutaneously in doses of 20 to 40 mg. However, relatively few physicians use it because of the rather severe and unpleasant side reactions which invariably occur after the administration of this drug. Its use may be dangerous and is therefore contraindicated in the presence of allergic asthma, anginal syndrome, and following myocardial infarction. It should never be given unless atropine is available for immediate intravenous use in the event that serious reactions occur. Mecholyl must be administered only *subcutaneously* and furthermore, because of the fall in blood pressure along with other untoward effects, Mecholyl should be given with the patient in the recumbent position.

If unsuccessful alone, the above mentioned drugs are frequently effective if carotid pressure or other vagal stimulation is applied fifteen minutes to one-half hour after the medications have been given.

A number of therapeutic agents have been recommended for the treatment of paroxysmal tachycardias. None has proved to be superior to those which have been discussed. An old-fashioned remedy is used by many practitioners; namely syrup of ipecac in doses of 4 to 8 cc. This will frequently abolish supraventricular tachycardias because of the vagal effect of inducing nausea and vomiting.

Paroxysmal Auricular Fibrillation

Although this arrhythmia may occur in normal individuals it is most commonly observed in the presence of organic heart disease. The transient or paroxysmal type of auricular fibrillation is usually benign and may occur without the patient's awareness. This is especially true when there are no structural changes in the heart.

Paroxysmal auricular fibrillation is a relatively common complication of hyperthyroidism and acute infections, such as pneumonia, even in the absence of structural heart changes. In patients with organic heart disease, including those with rheumatic carditis, fibrillation may precipitate acute heart failure or embolization. It therefore requires emergency treatment.

As with paroxysmal tachycardia, the initial treatment should include physical and mental rest obtained by means of a sedative, preferably a barbituric acid derivative. Morphine may be required in those patients with organic heart disease in whom heart failure may be precipitated by the arrhythmia.

Quinidine is usually effective in converting paroxysmal auricular fibrillation to normal sinus rhythm, and is considered by most clinicians to be the drug of choice for this purpose, regardless of the underlying type of heart disease. However, in the presence of a recent myocardial infarct, caution must be exercised in the use of quinidine, particularly if heart failure or embolism has occurred. There is no doubt that anticoagulant therapy has made this problem somewhat easier, since, with this treatment, the tendency for the deposition of mural thrombi and therefore of embolism can probably be diminished. Most clinicians digitalize patients who show signs of heart failure or who have a rapid ventricular rate as a result of auricular fibrillation. Quinidine is subsequently introduced if reversion to normal sinus rhythm is desired. In the presence of a recent myocardial infarct, or mitral stenosis, or in any other heart disorder in which embolism is likely to occur, anticoagulant treatment is indicated. It is imperative that good laboratory control be available when anticoagulants are used. There is no obvious contraindication to the use of quinidine simultaneously with digitalization or following it.[5] However, quinidine should never be employed in the presence of conduction defects or other evidence of digitalis intoxication. If there is no severe underlying heart disease and no factor which tends to perpetuate auricular fibrillation, such as hyperthyroidism or carditis, quinidine alone will usually restore normal sinus rhythm.

Quinidine sulfate, in doses of 0.4 Gm. given every two or three hours, will abolish most attacks of paroxysmal auricular fibrillation. If ineffectual after several doses, the dosage should be increased to 0.6 Gm. or higher. The drug should be continued until conversion of the arrhythmia has occurred or symptoms of intoxication appear. Among these are tinnitus, diminished hearing, vomiting, diarrhea or allergic manifestations. It is advisable to give no more than five successive doses in a single 24 hour period. If the patient is vomiting, or if any other condition precludes the oral administration of quinidine sulfate, quinidine may be administered intramuscularly with an initial dose of 0.6 Gm. It is wise to take repeated electrocardiograms during paren-teral quinidine administration and to be alert for the development of intraventricular or auriculoventricular conduction defects or other evidences of toxicity. Procaine amide (Pronestyl) may be effective in the conversion of this arrhythmia. The use and dosage of this drug will be discussed below under the treatment of ventricular tachycardia.

Quinacrine (atabrine) has recently been used in the treatment of paroxysmal auricular fibrillation.[6] It is reported to be as effective as quinidine in this arrhythmia and apparently has succeeded in the conversion of auricular fibrillation in cases where quinidine has failed. This would suggest that it may be of use for those patients who do not respond to or who may be sensitive to quinidine. Further clinical evaluation of this drug in the treatment of auricular fibrillation is necessary.

Paroxysmal Auricular Flutter

Most patients with this rhythm have some type of structural heart disease although, as in paroxysmal auricular fibrillation, it is some-times encountered in patients with normal hearts. Acute infections and hyperthyroidism are known to cause this arrhythmia.

In most cases of auricular flutter the patient is aware of the dis-turbance but is commonly in no great distress. However, heart failure may be present or may ensue, especially where the ventricular rate is rapid. While auricular flutter will occasionally respond to quinidine or to procaine amide, it is probably advisable to digitalize all patients with paroxysmal auricular flutter as soon as the arrhythmia is recog-nized. This is indicated particularly when there is a rapid ventricular rate, or when congestive failure is present or impending.

If flutter should occur in a patient with a recent myocardial infarct, and digitalis or quinidine is to be used, it is not necessary to employ anticoagulant therapy, as when auricular fibrillation occurs following infarction, since embolism rarely if ever takes place during flutter.[7]

When acute heart failure is associated with flutter, ouabain, lanatoside C, or Digoxin should be given intravenously, provided the patient has not received a digitalis preparation during the previous 14 days. If heart failure is not present or is of mild degree, digitalization may be accomplished orally over a period of a day or so, using the whole leaf of digitalis, or whatever glycoside the clinician prefers. Digitalis therapy usually results in one of the following eventualities: the flutter may be converted to fibrillation and remain as such; fibrillation may then be converted to normal sinus rhythm with quinidine, usually after digitalis has first been discontinued; fibrillation may revert to sinus rhythm spontaneously after withdrawal of digitalis without the necessity of using quinidine; or flutter may persist despite digitalization. In the latter instance, quinidine should be tried, as described under treatment of auricular tachycardia.

Ventricular Tachycardia

Ventricular tachycardia occurs, as a rule, in the presence of various structural changes in the heart, especially during the course of myocardial infarction. It is one of the most serious complications which may occur following infarction. Occasionally it is caused by digitalis intoxication, particularly in a patient with a seriously impaired myocardium. Uncommonly it occurs in a normal heart.

The presence of this arrhythmia should be suspected in any patient with heart disease who has a sudden change of heart rate to 160 to 200 or more beats per minute and which is basically regular in rhythm. It is well to remember that it can occur in complete heart block and that it may lead to bouts of ventricular fibrillation which, with ventricular tachycardia, may be a cause of Adams-Stokes seizures.

It is imperative that this rhythmic disturbance be abolished as soon as possible because of the ever present possibility that ventricular tachycardia may become ventricular fibrillation with fatal outcome. Treatment consists of absolute rest, induced, if necessary, by morphine administered subcutaneously or, in emergency, intravenously. At present, quinidine still remains the drug of choice in terminating this arrhythmia. A dose of 0.6 Gm. should be given orally and repeated every two hours until the rhythm reverts to one of sinus origin or until there are evidences of toxicity. These may first be evident in electrocardiograms, which ideally should be taken before each successive dose.

Electrocardiographic evidences of quinidine toxicity are conduction defects, chiefly with increase in QRS and the Q-T interval and lowering of the voltage. Recently several preparations (quinidine hydrochloride, quinidine dihydrochloride, quinidine lactate, quinidine gluconate, and quinidine sulfate) have become available which can be given *intramuscularly* without serious reactions. The recommended initial dose is 0.6 Gm. In desperate cases, quinidine may be used *intravenously* employing 0.6 Gm. diluted in 5 per cent glucose solution and given by the drip method. During quinidine administration, particularly when the drug is given parenterally, it is advisable to obtain serial electrocardiograms to follow the efficacy of treatment accurately and to watch for signs of toxicity. One authority[8] has recently reported the intravenous route of administration to have been successful in 20 out of 31 attacks. Despite this favorable result we should like to emphasize great caution in the intravenous administration of any form of quinidine because serious or fatal reactions may occur. It would be well if this route were used only when all other agents have failed and only if the patient is in a critical state.[9]

A new drug has recently made its appearance for use in the control of ventricular tachycardia. This is procaine amide hydrochloride (Pronestyl hydrochloride).[10] It appears to be sufficiently effective to offer promise. In a reported series, it failed in only two of 32 episodes of ventricular tachycardia.[11]

Preliminary observations of our own and others indicate that procaine amide is also effective in the treatment of supraventricular arrhythmias. These include paroxysmal auricular and nodal tachycardias, auricular fibrillation and auricular flutter. Procaine amide may be used as a substitute for quinidine; it may be tried in cases where quinidine treatment has been unsuccessful, or where there is intolerance to the latter drug. Like quinidine, procaine amide appears to be least effective when the arrhythmia has been of long standing.

Procaine amide may be employed both orally and intravenously; the latter route has been observed to cause a marked though transient fall in blood pressure. Nausea and vomiting have been noted occasionally as side effects but only where large doses are given orally. Clinical experience to date indicates procaine amide may be less toxic and more effective than quinidine in ventricular tachycardia. Evidence suggests that it is less dangerous when given intravenously than quinidine given by the same route. The dosage recommended for the administration of procaine amide is necessarily provisional at this time because of the limited number of cases which have been studied. The following dosage schedules are suggested: For oral use the drug is supplied in capsules of 250 mg. The oral route is advised with an initial dose of 1.25 Gm. This dose is frequently effective. If there has been no response and no evidence of toxicity, a second dose of 0.75 Gm. may be given in one hour. Further doses of 0.5 to 1.0 Gm. may be given at two to four hour intervals thereafter as required to terminate the aberrant rhythm. Procaine amide is supplied for parenteral (intravenous) use, in ampules of 10 cc., each cc. equivalent to 100 mg. The intravenous route is preferable only in patients who are unable to take oral medication or in acute emergencies, as when shock or failure are impending. The maximum rate of intravenous administration should be 200 mg. per minute, stopping the treatment when the rhythm reverts to normal, if there is any untoward effect or toxicity such as a fall in blood pressure, or when a total of 1 Gm. of procaine amide has been given. No more than 1 Gm. of the drug should be administered as a single intravenous dose. As in the use of parenteral quinidine it is helpful to take electrocardiograms, preferably with a direct-writing instrument, during intravenous administration. Procaine amide appears to have a quinidine-like action upon the heart. The toxic effects seen on the electrocardiogram are very similar to those of quinidine. They include prolongation of QRS and the Q-T interval and decrease in voltage. Rarely, ventricular tachycardia and ventricular fibrillation have resulted from procaine amide apparently because of too rapid administration or intravenous dosage in excess of 1 Gm.

In the treatment of ventricular tachycardias this new drug may make unnecessary trial with less effective agents, including magnesium sulfate, potassium chloride or Paredrine hydrobromide.

Although digitalis and its glycosides may, in toxic doses, produce ventricular tachycardia, the number of instances in which this occurs is probably small. The use of digitalis in the presence of ventricular tachycardia following myocardial infarction has recently been reviewed.[12] Symptoms, which could have been interpreted as being due to digitalis intoxication in three patients with ventricular tachycardia and heart failure, disappeared in spite of the continued use of digitalis.

The conclusions seem to indicate that digitalis may be used safely in the treatment of ventricular tachycardia when congestive heart failure is present. However, this requires further investigation before it can be completely accepted.

Complete Heart Block

This rhythmic disturbance may cause no symptoms. However, with the occurrence of an Adams-Stokes seizure, emergency treatment often becomes imperative. Dizziness and syncope, with or without convulsions, are the main symptoms of the syndrome.

Since the Adams-Stokes syndrome may be initiated by ventricular tachycardia or by ventricular fibrillation or may be caused by complete ventricular asystole, differential diagnosis must be decided by the electrocardiogram. The treatment is different depending upon which of the mechanisms is responsible. If the attack is due to ventricular tachycardia or fibrillation, quinidine or procaine amide appear to be the drugs of choice, used as outlined previously.

If an Adams-Stokes seizure is the result of asystole of the ventricles, epinephrine, 1 cc. (1:1000 dilution), is the drug to be used. It should be administered by injection into the heart. This may be followed by ephedrine sulfate, 25 mg. subcutaneously every four hours. If ventricular standstill continues, Paredrine hydrobromide[13] should be tried, also by injection into the heart. If cardiac standstill should occur while a patient is undergoing an operation, manual massage of the heart or direct electric stimulation of the ventricles of the exposed heart should be performed.[14]

If congestive heart failure occurs in the presence of complete heart block, digitalis should be administered. There is no contraindication to its use in this condition unless, of course, the arrhythmia is the result of digitalis intoxication.

Congestive Heart Failure

This condition is not infrequently an emergency in those instances where failure has appeared rapidly, or when a patient in congestive heart failure is in need of immediate surgical or obstetric care. Regardless of the type of heart disease, the basic principles of treatment are much the same. Management should be modified by the nature of the precipitating cause of the congestive heart failure. For example, if a myocardial infarct has induced heart failure it is considered advisable to use anticoagulant therapy, as well as such drugs as digitalis or one of its glycosides.

The greatest immediate benefit is accomplished by reducing the excessive burden carried by the impaired heart. This can be done by placing the patient at complete rest but not necessarily confined to bed. If there is considerable anxiety or pain, morphine should be administered subcutaneously or intravenously.

If there is no contraindication, particularly the use of digitalis within the previous two weeks, ouabain, Digoxin, or any rapidly acting digitalis preparation should be given intravenously, regardless of the heart rhythm. The initial dose of ouabain should be 0.5 mg., repeating 0.1 mg. every half to one hour or until therapeutic effect has been obtained, for a total of not more than 1 mg. Digoxin may be given with an initial dose of 0.5 mg., intravenously, followed by 0.25 mg. every four hours until a favorable response or a maximum of 1.5 mg. have been given. When using lanatoside C intravenously the first dose is 0.8 mg. followed by 0.4 mg. every two hours if needed to obtain a therapeutic response. Total dosage should generally not exceed 2.4 mg.

Acute Left Ventricular Failure

This emergency occurs most commonly in patients with the hypertensive type of heart disease. Left ventricular failure may occur also during or after operation, particularly if saline infusions or transfusions have been administered rapidly or in large quantity to a patient with structural heart disease. The prominent symptom is paroxysmal dyspnea; cough is also common. This initial phase may progress to pulmonary edema; then there is often expectoration of pink, frothy, watery sputum which may be raised in mouthfuls.

Morphine sulfate, 15 mg., combined with atropine sulfate, 0.6 mg., should immediately be administered hypodermically. If the urgency of the situation demands, morphine may be given intravenously. Nitroglycerin, when given early, seems to benefit some patients. The patient should be placed in Fowler's position or allowed to sit in a chair, where he will frequently be more comfortable than in bed. Oxygen therapy should be started as soon as possible. It should be administered by means of an oxygen mask metered for positive pressure (Meter Mask)[15] if available. With this method accurate control of pressure can be obtained by conducting the patient's expired air through water in a bottle calibrated in centimeters. It is advisable to begin with a pressure of 5 cm. of water which is gradually reduced to 1 cm. A concentration of 40 to 60 per cent oxygen with a volume flow of 8 to 10 liters a minute should be employed. Although masks are comfortable for some patients, they are objectionable to others. When discomfort prevents the administration of oxygen by mask, a change should be made to a tent, since this is an effective means of administrating 50 to 60 per cent oxygen. In order to obtain this concentration a maintenance flow of 10 to 12 liters per minute is necessary. Although a nasal catheter in the nasopharynx is as a rule more comfortable for long continued use, it is not as effective as the mask since the highest concentration possible by this method is only 40 per cent. A flow of 7 liters of oxygen a minute must be employed in order to maintain this concentration. Unfortunately, mouth breathing, which is quite prevalent, lowers the oxygen percentage in the air inhaled.

If the patient has not had any digitalis in the previous two weeks, ouabain, lanatoside C, Digoxin, or any other rapidly acting preparation, should be given intravenously. The dosage to be used has been described. However, if the patient is to undergo an emergency procedure such as an operation or an obstetric delivery, it is advisable to supplement and maintain the effects produced by a rapidly dissipated parenteral glycoside with the simultaneous administration of an oral digitalis preparation.[16] One advantage of this procedure is that rapid and complete digitalization is accomplished within 6 to 12 hours. The other is that it dispenses with the necessity of administering a digitalis preparation at repeated intervals during the first 24 hours. By this method, maintenance dosage may be started 24, or if necessary, 48 hours after initial digitalization which is performed as follows: a single dose of one of the rapidly acting glycosides is given parenterally. Simultaneously, a dose of one of the more slowly acting digitalis preparations is given orally, in a dosage depending on the estimated weight of the patient. Experience with this procedure has been most satisfactory, employing ouabain in a dose of 0.5 mg., intravenously, and the whole leaf tablet of digitalis (New York Heart Association Preparation, U.S.P. XIII) orally, in amounts ranging from 0.4 Gm. to 0.8 Gm., depending on body weight: 0.4 Gm. of digitalis leaf for weights to 125 pounds, 0.6 Gm. for weights of 125 to 175 pounds, and 0.8 Gm. for patients who weigh 175 pounds or more.

If for any reason a digitalis preparation cannot be used, aminophylline, 0.24 Gm., should be administered intravenously. It should be given slowly to avoid such reactions as headache, vertigo, palpitation, and possibly precordial pain or substernal oppression. It is best not to give this medication intramuscularly because of the intense local irritation which it usually causes. Suppositories of aminophylline are sometimes helpful as a substitute for, or as a supplement to, intravenous administration. The suppositories are supplied in 0.24 and 0.48 Gm. sizes. They are particularly useful in that they can be used by the patient at the onset of a bout of paroxysmal dyspnea and sometimes lessen the severity of the attack.

"Bloodless phlebotomy" may be an effective adjunct to treatment if pulmonary edema is accompanied by venous engorgement. The purpose of this procedure is to utilize the peripheral venous system as a reservoir, decrease the circulating blood volume, and thereby diminish the venous return to the heart. It is accomplished by applying tourniquets, preferably blood pressure cuffs, to all four extremities. Three of the cuffs are inflated at a time to a pressure slightly higher than the level of the patient's diastolic pressure. Release of each cuff is done in rotation every fifteen minutes to permit re-establishment of adequate blood flow. If this, and the measures outlined above, have not been successful in relieving the acute failure, phlebotomy, with the rapid withdrawal of at least 500 cc. of blood, should be performed.

Since the maintenance of an edema-free state is important, particularly in paroxysmal dyspnea or pulmonary edema, a mercurial diuretic should be administered intramuscularly or subcutaneously shortly after the measures described above have been initiated. A new mercurial diuretic, Thiomerin, which may be administered subcutaneously, intramuscularly, or intravenously, has been employed with excellent results.[17, 18] Based on ease of administration, degree of diuresis, and local tolerance, it is now considered by many to be the diuretic of choice.

Shock in Myocardial Infarction

Shock may be a complication of myocardial infarction. Its development is of very serious prognostic significance, as it is one of the main causes of death in the initial period following infarction.

The fall in blood pressure, which is often noted as part of a coronary attack, does not of itself constitute shock, even when systolic pressures of 90 mm. Hg or lower are present. Congestive failure, which not uncommonly occurs as a consequence of myocardial infarction, and which may be present concomitantly, should also not be confused with this condition.

Shock is identified by the following characteristic findings: The patient may be restless and apprehensive but he is more often in a semicomatose or comatose state. There is extreme pallor or cyanosis and the skin is cold and moist. The peripheral pulses are weak, thready or undetectable. The systolic pressure is usually 90 mm. Hg, or lower, and the pulse pressure is small; in patients who have previously manifested hypertension, the systolic pressure may be considerably higher than this figure.

Therapy should be based upon an understanding of the pathologic physiology which is responsible for the condition. Unfortunately, fundamental data concerning these mechanisms are inadequate and incomplete. There remains considerable controversy as to whether the primary mechanisms are cardiogenic or due to factors related to the vascular system. Because this process is not completely understood, plans of management of shock following myocardial infarction vary from the practice of "judicious neglect" to the use of a conglomeration of drugs and procedures based upon varied theoretic concepts.

The following are the most accepted measures in treatment: Elevation of the foot of the bed is of some value but is contraindicated if congestive failure is also present. High concentrations of oxygen administered by mask or tent should always be instituted as soon as possible. Artificial heating units should not be employed since burns may be easily produced in the presence of poor peripheral circulation and diminished sensory perception. Also, excessive sweating, due to external heat, may cause an additional loss of needed body fluids. The patient should, however, be covered with blankets sufficient to keep him comfortably warm. Bandaging the lower extremities from ankle to midthigh is thought by some to be of value. The use of the vasoconstrictor drugs is apparently increasing, although the question of their indication is controversial. These medications include Neosynephrine, ephedrine, Paredrine, and possibly norepinephrine. Paredrine is given in dosage of 10 to 20 mg. intramuscularly, or 5 to 10 mg. intravenously. The dosage of Neosynephrine is 5 mg. subcutaneously, or a maximum of 0.3 mg. may be given intravenously in dilute solution.

Morphine is indicated only if the patient is extremely restless, anxious, or in considerable pain. Otherwise it is contraindicated because the opiates depress pulmonary as well as tissue respiration and thereby tend to increase the degree of anoxia which is frequently found to be present.

It is known that if shock following myocardial infarction is treated with these measures alone, the mortality is still about 80 per cent. In view of this high mortality, more dynamic forms of therapy, if proved effective and not potentially too dangerous, would seem to be indicated. Until there is adequate understanding of the causative factors in this form of shock, we can only be guided in its treatment by experimental and clinical results following trial with various therapeutic measures.

Investigative studies on dogs appear to indicate that the early transfusion treatment of shock following coronary occlusion will improve failing myocardial contraction of the ischemic area and thereby probably increase cardiac output.[19] This work seems to justify the use of emergency measures directed at rapidly relieving acute shock following myocardial infarction, with the use of transfusions of blood or plasma and also with vasoconstrictor drugs.[19] Since hemoconcentration is frequently present, plasma transfusions may be preferable.

In recent years, some clinicians have advised the use of transfusions in this form of shock.[9] Reported clinical experiences with intravenous transfusion in the treatment of shock following myocardial infarction[20, 21] indicate that, while intravenous transfusions are not as yet of proved value, they have usually resulted in at least transient improvement. Where the treatment has failed it has appeared that larger, more frequent, or more rapidly administered transfusions might have reversed the shock picture or prevented recurrence. It has also been noted rather surprisingly that heart failure has rarely been produced by transfusions employed in this condition. Occasionally, indeed, where some degree of failure has been present at the time the transfusion was started, the signs have cleared following treatment.

On the basis of experience thus far, it appears that the use of transfusions following myocardial infarction is only definitely contraindicated when a high venous pressure, or marked pulmonary edema, is present.

Experimental studies[22] and preliminary clinical trials[23, 24] indicate that intra-arterial transfusions may be superior to intravenous transfusions in the treatment of this type of shock. Theoretic advantages of the intra-arterial, as compared with the intravenous route, are that intra-arterial transfusions effect a more prompt increase in blood pressure and probably of circulating blood volume. Consequently, there should be less danger of immediate overloading of the heart than with the use of larger intravenous transfusions. Experimental work on dogs in shock[22] has shown rapid retrograde perfusion of renal, coronary and cerebral arteries following arterial transfusion. In view of these considerations the use of intra-arterial transfusions of blood or plasma in the treatment of "coronary shock" warrants further investigation and evaluation.

Shock Following Pulmonary Embolism

Another form of shock which may be considered a cardiac emergency is that which frequently follows pulmonary embolism. Pulmonary emboli usually come from thrombi in the deep veins of the lower extremities or from the veins of the pelvis in surgical and obstetric patients. Symptoms are variable but in typical cases the patient suddenly becomes acutely dyspneic and cyanotic, is restless and anxious, complains of severe substernal oppression, and often there is rapid progress to shock and death. Differential diagnosis between pulmonary embolism and acute myocardial infarction may be difficult. History, x-ray, and especially the electrocardiogram are helpful in the diagnosis. Unfortunately, myocardial infarction is known to occur secondary to pulmonary embolism, in which circumstance evidences of both conditions will coexist. Prognosis of pulmonary embolism depends chiefly upon the size of the embolus, the severity of secondary reflex effects, and the promptness with which treatment directed at the relief of these factors is instituted.

In the treatment of this condition, oxygen should be given as soon as available. Morphine, combined with atropine, is administered if the patient is acutely dyspneic and is suffering from pain or anxiety. Vasodilator drugs are probably of considerable value in the presence of reflex vasospasm, but they should not be given if shock has developed. These medications include papaverine, 0.06 Gm., aminophylline, 0.48 Gm., and atropine, 0.6 mg., which are given by the intravenous route.

Anticoagulants have become one of the most important factors in reducing mortality and morbidity following pulmonary embolism. They are given to prevent propagation of thrombus in the pulmonary vessels and in an effort to control further embolization from the primary site. Heparin, because of its rapid action, should be given as early as possible. It is best administered intravenously in doses of 75 to 100 mg. which are repeated at six hour intervals until dicumarol or one of the more slowly acting anticoagulants, given simultaneously, has become fully effective. Proper laboratory control is, of course, essential. If further embolization occurs despite adequate anticoagulant therapy, bilateral femoral vein ligation and even ligation of the inferior vena cava may be indicated.

It should be kept in mind that pulmonary embolism can usually be prevented by the use of anticoagulants and the other prophylactic measures which should be employed in conditions where thromboembolic phenomena are apt to occur.

Cardiac Tamponade

Although this condition is not common it constitutes a serious emergency, which, if not treated promptly and properly, will invariably lead to death. The diagnosis of tamponade is missed with sufficient frequency to warrant a brief discussion to aid in its recognition.

Acute tamponade of the heart may occur following injury to the heart, to the pericardium, or to the great vessels. It results commonly from stab or gunshot wounds, but it may also complicate infections of the pericardium if there is considerable effusion. This is especially liable to occur in acute suppurative pericarditis. Rare, and invariably fatal, causes of tamponade are rupture of the heart following myocardial infarction, and retrograde progression of a so-called dissecting aneurysm of the aorta.

Patients with wounds and tamponade of the heart may be restless or in profound shock when first seen. The pulse is usually weak, thready, or imperceptible. Classically it is paradoxical in type. The blood pressure is commonly very low or unobtainable. The veins of the neck are distended. Heart sounds are generally distant or inaudible.

In the treatment of this condition aspiration of the pericardial space is usually indicated as an emergency measure to relieve tamponade. Early aspiration is also necessary because this blood clots rather rapidly and can be easily removed only soon after bleeding occurs. Fortunately, in many instances the bleeding does not recur and subsequent operation is not necessary.[25] However, if aspiration is not successful, or if signs of tamponade recur, open operation with suturing of the incised myocardium is indicated.

An aid in therapy which may help to prevent circulatory failure in acute pericardial tamponade is the rapid administration of intravenous infusions of saline, or of other intravenous solutions.[26, 27] The increase in venous pressure produced by this means will frequently overcome the resistance to the return of the blood to the right heart caused by tamponade. This increase may be sufficient to permit improvement in cardiac filling, and therefore of cardiac output. The result of this treatment is largely dependent upon whether the pericardial sac is able to stretch further. Intravenous infusion alone may aid in maintaining the circulation of the patient with tamponade. At least this appears to be a supportive measure which may be a valuable adjunct to aspiration or surgery.

A useful routine has been suggested[27] in the treatment of cardiac tamponade following stab wounds of the heart. The patient is given an infusion of saline solution and fluoroscoped immediately. If there are clinical and x-ray signs of tamponade, aspiration is performed immediately. The patient then receives a transfusion. If aspiration is unsuccessful or if the signs of pericardial tamponade recur after a successful aspiration, the heart is sutured.

Cardiac tamponade may also result from empyema secondary to acute suppurative pericarditis, or from large effusions such as are found in tuberculous pericarditis. Tamponade due to these causes produces circulatory failure of the same type as that observed in patients with stab wounds of the heart. It is treated by aspiration or by surgery with open drainage if aspiration is inadequate. Penicillin or other antibiotics may be of value when instilled directly into the pericardial sac in suppurative pericarditis following initial aspiration or surgical drainage. This is usually supplemented by systemic antibiotic therapy.

Acknowledgments

This work is from the Third and Fourth (New York University) Medical Divisions, Bellevue Hospital, and the Lenox Hill Hospital, New York, N. Y.

References

[1] Stewart, H. J.: How to use digitalis. M. Clin. North America *34:* 649, 1950.

[2] Weisberger, A. S., and Feil, H.: Lanatoside C in the treatment of persistent paroxysmal auricular tachycardia. Am. Heart J. *34:* 871, 1947.

[3] Rose, O. A., Batterman, R. C., and DeGraff, A. C.: Clinical studies on digoxin: a purified digitalis glycoside. Am. Heart J. *24:* 435, 1942.

[4] DeGraff, A. C.: Digitalis and cardiac glycosides in congestive heart failure. M. Clin. North America *34:* 663, 1950.

[5] DiPalma, J. R., and Schults, J. E.: Antifibrillatory drugs. Medicine *29:* 123, 1950.

[6] Gertler, M. M., and Yohalem, S. B.: The effect of atabrine (quinacrine hydrochloride) on cardiac arrhythmias. Am. Heart J. *37:* 79, 1949.

[7] Askey, J. M.: Auricular flutter in association with myocardial infarction; its prognosis and management. Am. J. Med. *6:* 453, 1949.

[8] Armbrust, C. A., Jr. and Levine, S. A.: Paroxysmal ventricular tachycardia. A study of 107 cases. Circulation *1:* 28, 1950.

[9] de la Chapelle, C. E.: The management of the acute episode in coronary occlusion. Bull. New York Acad. Med. *19:* 201, 1943.

[10] Mark, L. C., Berlin, I., Kayden, H. J., Rovenstine, E. A., Steele, J. M., and Brodie, B. B.: The action of procaine amide on ventricular arrhythmia (abstract). J. Pharmacol. & Exper. Therap. *98:* 21, 1950.

[11] ——, Kayden, H. J., Steele, J. M., Cooper, J. R., Berlin, I., Rovenstine, E. A., and Brodie, B. B.: The physiological disposition and cardiac effects of procaine amide. J. Pharmacol. & Exper. Therap. *102:* 5, 1951.

[12] Gilson, J. S., and Schemm, F. R.: The use of digitalis in spite of the presence of ventricular tachycardia. Circulation *2:* 287, 1950.

[13] Herrmann, G.: Circulatory mechanism disorders; recognition and management of common sudden disturbances. J. Missouri M. A. *37:* 421, 1940.

[14] Beck, C. S.: Resuscitation for cardiac standstill and ventricular fibrillation occurring during operation. Am. J. Surg. *54:* 273, 1936.

[15] Committee on Public Health Relations of the New York Acad. Med.: Standards of effective administration of inhalational therapy. J. A. M. A. *144:* 25, 1950.

[16] Batterman, R. C., Rose, O. A., and DeGraff, A. C.: Combined use of ouabain and digitalis in treatment of congestive heart failure. Am. Heart J. *20:* 443, 1940.

[17] ——: The treatment of congestive heart failure with mercurial diuretics. M. Clin. North America *34:* 629, 1950.

[18] STEWART, H. J., McCOY, H. I., SHEPHARD, E. M., AND LUCKEY, E. H.: Experience with thiomerin, a new mercurial diuretic. Circulation *1:* 502, 1950.

[19] CORDAY, E., BERGMAN, H. C., SCHWARTZ, L. L., SPRITZLER, R. J., AND PRINZMETAL, M.: Studies on the coronary circulation. IV. The effect of shock on the heart and its treatment. Am. Heart J. *37:* 560, 1949.

[20] SAMPSON, J. J., AND SINGER, I. M.: Plasma and blood infusions following myocardial infarction. Am. Heart J. *38:* 54, 1949.

[21] EPSTEIN, F. H., AND RELMAN, A. S.: Transfusion treatment of shock due to myocardial infarction. New England J. Med. *241:* 889, 1949.

[22] PAGE, I. H.: On certain aspects of the nature and treatment of oligemic shock. Am. Heart J. *38:* 161, 1949.

[23] WEISMAN, S. J.: The treatment of shock in acute myocardial infarction; a review. Am. Practitioner *1:* 1078, 1950.

[24] Personal observations.

[25] BLALOCK, A., AND RAVITCH, N. N.: A consideration of the non-operative treatment of cardiac tamponade resulting from wounds of the heart. Surgery *14:* 157, 1943.

[26] COOPER, F. W., JR., STEAD, E. A., JR., AND WARREN, J. V.: The beneficial effect of intravenous infusions in acute pericardial tamponade. Ann. Surg. *120:* 822, 1944.

[27] WARREN, J. V., BRANNON, E. S., STEAD, E. A., JR., AND MERRILL, A. J.: Pericardial tamponade from stab wound of the heart and pericardial effusion or empyema: A study utilizing the method of right heart catheterization. Am. Heart J. *31:* 418, 1946.

Surgery for Mitral Stenosis. A Review of Progress

By Edward F. Bland, M.D.

THE PAST five years have witnessed a widespread renewal of interest in operations for mitral stenosis. Our surgical colleagues have pushed forward with courage, skill, and notable success, their efforts to relieve the obstructed mitral orifice. It is the purpose of this report to review briefly the background of this revival, to summarize the more recent developments and, with the cooperation of those most concerned, to appraise the results and the risks involved. Our interest is primarily from the point of view of the patient and his physician; surgical technics are not our concern.

Early Contributions

A capitulation of the attempts in the past to break down the barrier of stenotic valves is a fascinating exposition of boldness, persistence, and futility. Until the turn of the century the prevailing views as to the surgical sanctity of the heart were epitomized by the renowned Billroth in 1883: "Let no man who hopes to retain the respect of his medical brethren dare to operate on the human heart."

However, the advent of asepsis, experimental laboratories, and another century opened new vistas. It was Sir Thomas Lauder Brunton (of amyl nitrite fame) who proposed in 1902 the possibility of surgical intervention for mitral stenosis. Although this precipitated a vigorous and somewhat sarcastic editorial in the next issue of the London Lancet of that year,[31] it served to stimulate further the experimental approach which had already demonstrated in animals the feasibility of such a procedure (Klebs, 1876), and led to the subsequent studies of MacCallum (1906), Cushing and Branch (1908), Bernheim (1909), and Schepelmann (1912).

Thus was the stage set for the first attempt in a human being by

Doyen in 1913. Instead of a patient with mitral stenosis, he chose a young woman of 20 with congenital pulmonary stenosis, and he attempted to relieve the obstruction with a tenotome knife passed through the right ventricle. The patient expired a few hours later and necropsy revealed a tubular narrowing of the conus (as is often the case) rather than a localized stenosis of the valve.

A year later Tuffier (1914) exposed the heart of a young man with advanced aortic stenosis. It was his intention to insert a knife above the aortic ring and incise the stenosed valve, but during the operation this plan was abandoned. Instead, dilatation of the stenosed orifice was accomplished by invaginating the wall of the aorta with the forefinger. The patient survived and was reported living and possibly improved 10 years later.

Thereafter another decade elapsed and the extensive experience with cardiac wounds in World War I accrued before further attempts were forthcoming.

In 1923 Cutler and Levine reported the first case of a successful section of the valve for advanced mitral stenosis.[24] The patient, a girl of 11 years, had been observed for eight months at the House of the Good Samaritan (Boston) with recurring episodes of acute dyspnea and hemoptysis, and because of the increasing gravity of her symptoms she was transferred to the Peter Bent Brigham Hospital for surgery. A tenotome knife was passed through the left ventricle and an attempt made to incise each cusp of the obstructing mitral ring. Although the postoperative state was critical, the patient survived, but the signs of mitral stenosis persisted; the diastolic murmur was slightly altered and there was a prolongation of her systolic murmur. She lived four and a half years after operation, but her activities were seriously limited and she required hospitalization on several occasions for rest and treatment. She finally succumbed with bronchopneumonia and extensive congestion of the lungs.

Necropsy revealed moderate stenosis of the valve, but the orifice admitted a bougie 4 cm. in circumference. The site of the previous incision was easily recognized by a defect in the thickened rolled edge of the valve ring joined towards the base by a thinner membrane-like structure (fig. 1). There seemed no doubt the orifice had been enlarged by the operation. Furthermore, there was no suggestion of an overgrowth of scar tissue in the healing process. This is a key case: it not only represents the first survivor of valve section but the subsequent four and a half years of life also provide an indication of the favorable type of valve healing hoped for in those now being submitted to surgery.

During the next five years (1923–28) Cutler and his associates undertook a somewhat similar procedure in six additional patients: none survived.[23] Allen, also in 1923, attempted to approach the valve through the left atrium with a cardioscope devised by Allen and Graham,[6] but the patient succumbed during the procedure.[5]* Souttar (1925) successfully dilated the mitral ring by finger and his patient survived (a forerunner of the present most favored procedure), but Pribram's attempt (1925) with a valvulotome through the left ventricle ended fatally on the fifth day.

Thus, during the 1920's 10 patients with mitral stenosis were subjected to valve section or digital dilatation as follows:

> Cutler and associates (section)   7 (1 survived)
> Allen (cardioscope)   1
> Souttar (dilatation)   1 (survived)
> Pribram (section)   1

The 80 per cent mortality was discouraging. However, in spite of this unfavorable experience, interest at the laboratory level continued, and between 1929 and 1932 Powers was successful in producing in dogs gross deformity of the mitral cusps by electrical coagulation followed by infection with intravenous inoculations of *Streptococcus viridans*.[50] Later healing in those who survived yielded a scarred valve with an element of stenosis. Subsequent valvulotomy led to acute cardiac dilatation and failure in the majority of the animals.[51] From these experiments he concluded that the abrupt creation of mitral regurgita-

---

* It is of interest, particularly for historical accuracy, to note that since the earlier reports of Cutler and Beck,[23] and including the more recent ones of Karken,[40] of Bailey,[8] and of others,[10] reference to this case operated upon in 1923 has been erroneously cited as "Allen, D. S., and Graham, E. A.: J. A. M. A. September 23, 1922," and "Allen, D. S.: Arch. Surg. January, 1924."

A careful check of these two references reveals no mention whatsoever of a human case. In view of this discrepancy and the obvious error perpetuated through almost a quarter of a century, and in response to a personal communication from the author, Dr. Evarts A. Graham kindly supplied the correct reference to the original report by Dr. Duff S. Allen.[5]

tion was a hazardous procedure which in man might likewise lead to acute decompensation and death.

Clinical support for this deduction was inferred from the remarkable case recorded by Adam (1927) of perforation of the anterior leaflet of the mitral valve by a bullet in a young man of 19 who attempted suicide but survived. He was left with the sign of pure mitral regurgi-

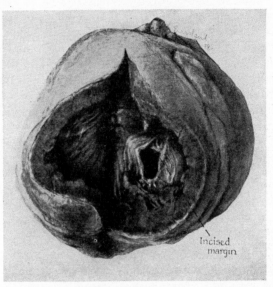

FIG. 1. Photograph of the mitral valve of Cutler and Levine's patient who lived four and one-half years after valvulotomy. The site of incision was easily recognized by a defect in the thickened rolled edge of the valve ring joined at the base by the thinner membrane-like structure. (Cutler and Beck: Arch. Surg. *18:* 403, 1929.)

tation—a loud blowing systolic murmur at the cardiac apex. He lived 10 years, but his course was marked by progressive cardiac enlargement, auricular fibrillation, chronic congestive failure, and death. A photograph of this unique specimen is reproduced in figure 2, since, as in Cutler and Levine's case, it gives a clue to the type of healing which occurs following valve trauma (and surgery). Healing around the defect had been accompanied by only minimal thickening of the adjacent valve substance. It is of further interest that as a result of regurgitation all the heart chambers in this case were greatly hypertrophied and dilated.

Thus it is understandable that these combined clinical and laboratory failures temporarily discouraged further attempts at valve surgery until after World War II. In the interim, from a combination of circumstances, there evolved slowly an attitude of renewed confidence where heretofore the dismay of former failures had prevailed.

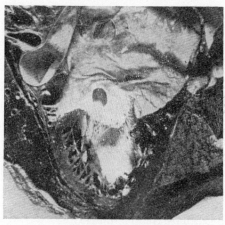

FIG. 2. Photograph of perforation of the anterior leaflet of the mitral valve (bullet wound) in Adam's patient who survived 10 years with pure mitral regurgitation. (Adam: Ztschr. Kreislaufforsch. *19:* 313, 1927.)

Notable in this connection were the remarkable results obtained in the correction of congenital defects, as well as the favorable experience with cardiac wounds in another world war—this time with the actual removal of missiles from the heart cavities—and finally, there emerged a new generation of dynamic surgeons, fully fortified with catheterization data[21, 36] and hydraulic formulas.[35] The inevitable outcome was a more sustained and successful attack upon the obstructing valve.

Collateral Procedures

Discouraged by the prohibitive mortality of the earlier efforts to relieve mitral stenosis by a direct approach, others sought an indirect solution to the problem.

A special challenge was presented by those patients with high grade stenosis, little or no cardiac enlargement, and recurring (sometimes fatal) attacks of acute pulmonary congestion and hemorrhage. Their disability clearly involves extreme pulmonary hypertension behind an obstructed valve outlet, secondary alterations in the lungs, and a strong right ventricle. Under conditions of stress, tachycardia and increased blood volume the augmented activity of the hypertrophied right ventricle floods the lungs whose outlet is fixed by the narrowed mitral orifice. Under these circumstances pulmonary edema and hemorrhage are inevitable. It is an acute increment in the already excessive pulmonary pressure which is responsible for this vascular crisis within the lungs (fig. 3). Medical measures (digitalis, diuretics, and diets), although helpful, are ultimately ineffective in dealing with this clinical paradox.

Two clues exist which suggest that help might be available for them outside the heart. In 1926 Jarotzky called attention to the apparent protection afforded the lungs in patients with mitral stenosis who had a congenital atrial septal defect (Lutembacher's syndrome). The protective action of this defect in lessening pulmonary hypertension and congestion has been substantiated by clinical observation,[11, 16] and by catheter studies.[27] Jarotzky suggested that the surgical creation of such a defect might be helpful, as did O'Farrell in 1938. This was actually accomplished by Harken in 1948 but has now been abandoned in favor of the direct operation upon the valve.[40]

Another clue in a different direction is presented by the remarkably dilated bronchial veins in patients with longstanding mitral stenosis—an attempt by nature to provide an outlet from the congested pulmonary bed into the systemic veins.[32] Thus, in those whose pulmonary syndrome is characterized by massive hemorrhage from these dilated varices (on occasion up to 500 cc.), the accompanying edema is often strikingly relieved or actually aborted. It is unfortunate that this natural protective mechanism sometimes leads to fatal exsanguination.[49]

In 1946, with these facts in mind, Bland and Sweet decided that a vent from the high pressure area of the left atrium or adjacent pulmonary veins into a systemic vein might offer relief to these patients. At that time an extracardiac shunt seemed less risky than either an intracardiac septal defect or a direct operation upon the valve. After two more years of deliberation and study the operation was successfully performed (March 1948) on a 17 year old girl.[16, 17, 59] An anastomosis was effected between a branch of the right inferior pulmonary vein and the azygos vein (fig. 4). A vigorous diversion of blood from the pulmonary circuit into the systemic vein ensued. Direct measurements of left intra-atrial pressure in later cases confirmed the hope that a significant lessening of tension would result. The subsequent course of this patient was so remarkable, and the animal experiments of Swan were so encouraging, that during the following two years

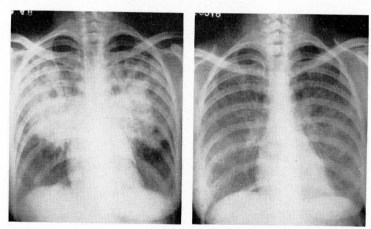

FIG. 3. Acute and near fatal pulmonary edema in a woman aged 24 with advanced mitral stenosis but with little or no cardiac enlargement. *Left.* Roentgenogram on entry showing extensive edema of the lungs with characteristic butterfly distribution. *Right.* Roentgenogram three days after rapid subsidence of the edema.

(1948–49) 12 patients with recurring severe pulmonary edema were likewise operated upon, and more recently two additional patients have had this procedure. Certain physiologic data assembled at the time of operation are shown in table 1. It is to be noted that the pressure by direct measurement in the left atrium was from four to five times normal in all instances, and upon release of the shunt there usually occurred within a few moments a prompt drop of approximately 80 mm. of saline (unpublished data, Bland and Sweet, 1951).

The later course of this group has been of special interest. Fully half have had striking and continued relief from pulmonary edema, several were much benefited for one to two years but are now beginning to have milder recurrences of their previous trouble (suggesting a possible closure of the shunt), a few had only questionable benefit, and three succumbed within a few days of the procedure.

As was emphasized originally by the authors, this procedure is at best a compromise and not a cure. It was designed only for those with relatively small strong hearts as a protection to the lungs.

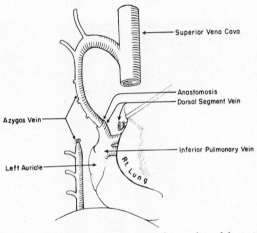

FIG. 4. Diagram of the pulmonary-azygos shunt viewed from the right side. The lung has been retracted forward. Oxygenated blood from the high pressure pulmonary circuit escapes backward through the anastomosis to the low pressure systemic bed distending the azygos vein to its juncture with the superior vena cava. (Bland and Sweet: J. A. M. A. *140:* 1259, 1949.)

In France, d'Allaines and associates, unaware of this earlier work in Boston, performed a somewhat similar procedure (January 1949) and subsequently operated on 16 additional patients with encouraging results in the majority,[2, 3] but they have now shifted to the direct approach (as have Bland and Sweet) as a more promising and less difficult operation.[43]

These purely palliative measures of the past three years have now been overshadowed and quite properly replaced in large measure by the direct attack upon the mitral valve. The remarkable improvement in technic and the consequent lessening of the risk have rendered other methods less attractive and somewhat obsolete, but nevertheless useful, perhaps, under special circumstances where complicating aortic valve disease (regurgitation) already places a strain upon the left ventricle.

TABLE 1.—*Measurements made at operation by means of a needle passed into the left atrium (usually through a pulmonary vein) and recorded in millimeters of saline before and after release of the shunt. (Bland and Sweet, unpublished data, 1951.)*

ADVANCED MITRAL STENOSIS

LEFT AURICULAR PRESSURE

Direct Measurements at Operation
(Normal = $100 \pm$ mm. H_2O)

CASE	CLOSED	SHUNT	OPEN
1. O.C.	460		
3. R.O.	425		390
4. D.G.			450
5. A.P.	530		370
6. E.R.	460		370
7. L.G.	480		370
8. E.J.	300		180
9. E.P.	475 ?		475
10. A.O.	370		350
12. R.J.	440		
13. T.R.	510		430
AVERAGE OF 8 COMPLETED CASES	447	(80)	367

Direct Operations

Concurrently with the foregoing developments, a more aggressive attack upon the valve itself by several groups has yielded remarkable results, a colorful glossary of terms (valvuloplasty, commissurotomy, finger-fracture, and stenotomy) and, in certain quarters, even a new philosophy which intimates that all patients with mitral stenosis should have their valves split.

In the forefront, and a brilliant exponent of this resurgent interest in valve surgery, was H. G. Smithy, Jr. His untimely death in 1948 at 34 was a tragic loss—he was himself a victim of aortic stenosis.

Through the continuing efforts of Harken in Boston, of Bailey in Philadelphia, of Blalock in Baltimore, and of Brock in London, as well as of others elsewhere, enough data have now accumulated to warrant an appraisal of the present status and future promise of the direct approach. I am indebted to these surgeons and in particular to their medical associates* for permitting me to pool their results for the purpose of this report. Minor differences of opinion exist as to technics and indications, but there is wholehearted agreement as to the immediate benefits to be expected, of respect for the risks involved and of the uncertainties of the future.

In regard to technic, all agree that the approach through the left atrial appendage is safest and surest. Most surgeons prefer digital dilatation, with "finger-fracture" when possible, as less risky than incision in a blind field with a valvulotome. It is clear, however, that each method has a place. In general, calcified valves fracture more readily than heavily scarred and gristly structures. Unfortunately, a few are encountered for which neither method is adaptable. In the author's clinic the following situations have rendered operation either impossible or prohibitively risky: (1) a markedly gristly, funnel-shaped valve, impossible to fracture or to incise successfully even at the autopsy table (postmortem case); (2) an abnormally narrow communication (less than 1 cm. diameter) between the appendage and atrial cavity, plus structural deformity rendering the alternative approach through a pulmonary vein too dangerous; (3) a high degree of mitral regurgitation evident at operation in spite of "unequivocal" clinical and catheter evidence of high-grade pure mitral stenosis.

Figure 5 illustrates the most favored procedure, so-called "finger-fracture valvuloplasty" (Harken). It has been emphasized by Harken and his associates, and substantiated by others, that incision in the region of the anterior cusp is followed by far greater regurgitation than is an operation on the posterior cusp (selective insufficiency) or resection of the immobilizing commissure bridges.[40] Bailey and his group prefer incision in the region of the obliterated commissures which favors (in agreement with Harken) less regurgitation and more effec-

* I am especially indebted for personal communications concerning the medical aspects of the operated cases from Drs. E. Cowles Andrus (Baltimore), Maurice Campbell (London), George C. Griffith (Los Angeles), and Prof. J. Lenègre (Paris).

tive valve function—so-called "commissurotomy" (Durant), as shown in figure 6.[8, 33, 34] More recently a less descriptive but more inclusive term, "stenotomy," has been suggested for both procedures (Alroy).

An ingenious and different approach has been undertaken by Murray. A cardioscope is passed through the left ventricle, and the mitral valve is resected. In order to compensate for the resulting regurgitation, a sling-like structure composed of a section of vein,

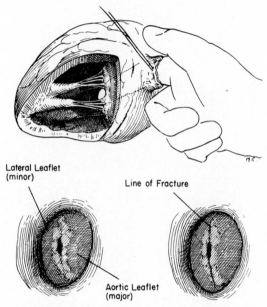

Lateral Leaflet
(minor)

Line of Fracture

Aortic Leaflet
(major)

FIG. 5. Diagram of finger-fracture valvuloplasty. The index finger is passed through the left auricular appendage and left auricle to reach the mitral orifice. (Courtesy of Dr. Dwight E. Harken, 1951.)

everted and supported with a length of tendon, is suspended on the ventricular side of the orifice for a ball-valve action. Of 10 patients, there were eight survivors. It would seem, however, that this procedure is too complicated and too unphysiologic to offer promise.

For the special purpose of this report a survey of the experiences in selected centers in this country and abroad indicates that during the past three years, 352 patients with mitral stenosis have been operated upon, and from collateral reports of operations elsewhere it is quite likely that the total now approaches 500 cases.

In table 2 are summarized the results furnished the author (mostly as of May 1951) from seven centers. The 352 cases include the early

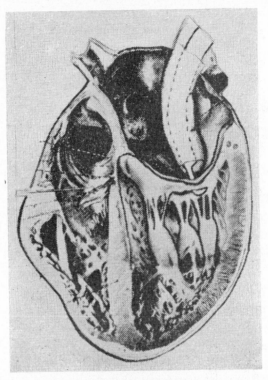

Fig. 6. Diagram of commissurotomy. The right index finger bearing the commissurotomy knife has been inserted through the left auricular appendage and the hooked blade engaged on the lateral commissure. (Glover, Bailey and O'Neill: J. A. M. A. *144:* 1049, 1950.)

and hence most unfavorable types; thus the mortality figures are weighted in an unfavorable direction. With rapid improvement in technics and a more discriminating selection of patients, there has been a gratifying improvement in the results, so that now a fair estimate indicates a 10 to 15 per cent operative risk for those patients with relatively slight to moderate cardiac enlargement but with advanced mitral stenosis and severe pulmonary hypertension, and a correspondingly greater risk for those with larger and weaker hearts. The further hazard of postoperative embolism, although often nonfatal, remains a distressing aftermath for a few (6 per cent).

An early and dramatic improvement has occurred in the majority of patients. Further clinical observation and catheter studies support the substantial benefits predicted from the early improvement.[26, 29]

TABLE 2.—*Operations for Mitral Stenosis**

	Cases	Mortality	Embolism	Improved
Bailey et al.[9] (Philadelphia)....	165	17 (10.3%)	9 (5.4%)	"majority"
Harken et al.[38] (Boston).......	62	17 (27.4%)	4 (6.4%)	"majority"
Brock et al.[19] (London)........	50	8 (16.0%)	2 (4.0%)	37 (74.0%)
Blalock et al.[14] (Baltimore)....	30	2 (6.6%)	1 (3.3%)	26 (86.9%)
Longmire et al.[44] (Los Angeles)	25	4 (16.0%)	4 (16.0%)	"most"
Brantigan[18] (Baltimore)........	12	3 (25.0%)	1 (8.3%)	7 (58.3%)
Author's series (Boston)†......	8	2 (25.0%)	0	6 (75.0%)
Totals.....................	352	53 (15.0%)	21 (6.0%)	

* As of approximately May 1951.

† Operations by Drs. J. G. Scannell and R. Warren.

Selection of Cases

The selection of patients for either of these formidable procedures must of necessity rest largely with the internist and cardiologist. This aspect has been emphasized recently by Harken and co-workers.[39] I am indebted to the internists intimately associated with the surgeons listed in table 2 for their opinion and criteria in the selection of patients.

In general it is agreed that the most suitable cases are those with a high degree of mitral stenosis with little or no evident regurgitation, and with unmistakable signs and symptoms of pulmonary engorgement (dyspnea, cough, pulmonary edema, or hemoptysis). The smaller the heart, the better the outlook. Those with large hearts and chronic congestive failure are poor risks and are unlikely to benefit significantly from surgery. Auricular fibrillation or previous embolism increase the hazards slightly but do not constitute contraindications per se. It is unlikely except in special instances that worthwhile benefit can accrue for patients beyond 50 years of age.

There are two absolute contraindications to surgery: active rheumatic carditis and bacterial endocarditis. Measurable strain on the left ventricle from aortic regurgitation (less often stenosis) or from mitral regurgitation renders operations on the mitral valve doubly dangerous. In special cases where, in spite of these latter complications, the patient's life is being threatened by recurring pulmonary edema, a pulmonary-azygos shunt may offer a reasonable compromise. We have recently undertaken this successfully as an alternative in a patient with considerable aortic regurgitation.

A further attempt to classify patients into subgroups for assessment for surgery may ultimately prove useful, but at the moment it is somewhat unsatisfactory and controversial. For the present the general principles outlined above seem safest.

The high incidence of Aschoff bodies (up to 25 per cent) noted in biopsies of the atrial appendage has been a surprising finding and out of line with clinical evidence of rheumatic activity. In view of the scant evidence under these circumstances of clinical rheumatic activity and the absence of significant postoperative reactivation, there is need for a further critical review of these clinical-pathologic relationships and perhaps some modification in our present concepts of "activity."

In concluding this review, it is with awesome admiration that one recounts the remarkable progress of the past five years made by our surgical colleagues. In the face of the dramatic improvement after operation in these often desperately ill patients, the enthusiasm of the moment is understandable, and the desire to extend these possible benefits to those not yet in need of help is tempting, especially since they present to the surgeon more favorable operative risks. In this connection, however, it is timely to emphasize that mitral stenosis is not always a progressive lesion and patients with lesser degrees of deformity may attain a comfortable old age. The long term observations of Bland and Jones on 1000 children followed for 20 years after rheumatic fever reveal the development of mitral stenosis in 117 patients. Of this group during the two decades of follow-up, only 12 have progressed to a state of disabling pulmonary hypertension with acute pulmonary edema and hemorrhage (now mostly in the third decade). Encouraging also in the older age group (from 30 to 40) are the factual data of Grant on the after-history of 1000 soldiers invalided from the British Army after World War I with valvular heart disease. During the 10 year period of observation he found that in those with mitral stenosis:

"The prognosis in cases with signs of early stenosis is good and in them exercise tolerance is best and cardiac enlargement least; about half live uneventfully and unchanged, only a small proportion, about 5 per cent, develop auricular fibrillation and congestive failure, and about 10 per cent die within 10 years. In the presence of great cardiac enlargement and congestive failure the prognosis is bad, very few cases displaying these signs survive the 10 years; the average of life is four to five years."

Further data on the adult age groups by decades are needed and will soon be available, but for the moment a formidable operation upon the mitral valve had best be reserved for those in need of relief and the benefits to date justify the risk involved. On the contrary, for those with little or no disability the operation seems illogical and ill advised. The possible creation in this group of an uncertain element of regurgitation and the hazards of premature auricular fibrillation and embolism render the procedure unacceptable as a purely preventive measure. The ultimate solution for the majority of these patients is more subtle than the simple correction of a mechanical defect: their problem involves also a diseased myocardium, and their fate is inexorably linked with the vagaries of their rheumatic state.

Summary

The renewed interest in surgery for mitral stenosis is reviewed and the progress of the past five years summarized. The present status of the indirect operation (pulmonary-azygos shunt) is discussed, and the notable advances with the direct attack (finger-fracture valvuloplasty and commissurotomy) have been brought up to date (May 1951) by means of a survey of selected centers here and abroad.

Detailed information is available on 352 patients who have had an operation on the mitral valve. It is quite likely that the total now approaches 500 cases.

The over-all operative mortality has been 15 per cent. Post-operative embolism occurred in 6 per cent. Clinical improvement in the majority has been prompt and striking, and this has been fully supported by catheterization data. An appraisal of the more remote effects must await the passage of time.

Those most likely to benefit are patients under the age of 50 with only slight to moderate cardiac enlargement who are nevertheless seriously limited by pulmonary hypertension and congestion.

A formidable procedure of this magnitude should be reserved for those in trouble; it has no place in the management of patients with little or no disability.

ACKNOWLEDGMENT

This work is from the Massachusetts General Hospital, Boston, Mass.

REFERENCES

[1] ADAM, A.: Ueber die traumatischen Veranderungen gesunder Klappen des Herzens. Ztschr. f. Kreislaufforsch. *19:* 313, 1927.

[2] D'ALLAINES, F., LENÈGRE, J., DUBOST, C., MATHIVAT, A., AND SCÉBAT, L.: L'anastomose veine pulmonaire—veine azygos dans le rétrécissement mitral à propos d'un cas opéré avec succès. (1) Bull. et mém. soc. méd. hôp. Paris *65:* 512, 1949. (2) Arch. mal. coeur *42:* 456, 1949.

[3] ——, ——, ——, SCÉBAT, L., AND MATHIVAT, M.: L'anastomose veineuse azygo-pulmonaire dans le traitement du rétrécissement mitral oedemateux. Cardiologia *15:* 266, 1949.

[4] ALLEN, D. S.: Intracardiac surgery. Arch. Surg. *8:* 317, 1924.

[5] ——: Le traitement chirurgical de la stenose mitrale. Arch. franco-belges de chir. *28:* 394, 1925.

[6] ——, AND GRAHAM, E. A.: Intracardiac surgery: a new method. J. A. M. A. *79:* 1028, 1922.

[7] ALROY, MICHAEL: Surgery of mitral disease. Lancet *1:* 1369, 1951.

[8] BAILEY, C. P.: The surgical treatment of mitral stenosis (mitral commissurotomy). Dis. Chest *15:* 377, 1949.

[9] BAILEY, C. P.: Personal communication, April 1951.

[10] BAKER, C., BROCK, R. C., AND CAMPBELL, M.: Valvulotomy for mitral stenosis. Report of six successful cases. Brit. M. J. *1:* 1283, 1950.

[11] BEDFORD, D. E., PAPP, C., AND PARKINSON, J.: Atrial septal defect. Brit. Heart J. *3:* 37, 1941.

[12] BERNHEIM, B. M.: Experimental surgery of mitral valve. Bull. Johns Hopkins Hosp. *20:* 107, 1909.

[13] BILLROTH, T., quoted from Jeger, E.: Die Chirurgie der Blutgefasse und des Herzens. Berlin, A. Hirschwald, 1913. P. 295.

[14] BLALOCK, A.: Personal communication from Dr. E. C. Andrus (Blalock, A. and Bing, R.), May 1951.

15 BLAND, E. F., AND JONES, T. D.: Rheumatic fever and rheumatic heart disease: A twenty-year report on 100 patients followed since childhood. Circulation *4:* 836, 1951.

16 ——, AND SWEET, R. H.: A venous shunt for marked mitral stenosis. Mass. General Hospital, Case 53. Am. Pract. *2:* 756, 1948.

17 ——, AND ——: A venous shunt for advanced mitral stenosis. J. A. M. A. *140:* 1259, 1949.

18 BRANTIGAN, O. C.: Personal communication, July 1951.

19 BROCK, R. C.: Personal communication from Baker, C., Brock, R. C., Campbell, M., and Wood, P., April 1951.

20 BRUNTON, T. L.: Preliminary note on possibility of treating mitral stenosis by surgical methods. Lancet *1:* 352, 1902.

21 COURNAND, A.: Some aspects of the pulmonary circulation in normal man and in chronic cardiopulmonary disease. Circulation *2:* 641, 1950.

22 CUSHING, H., AND BRANCH, J. R. B.: Experimental and clinical notes on chronic valvular lesions in the dog and their possible relation to further surgery of the cardiac valves. J. M. Research *12:* 471, 1908.

23 CUTLER, E. C., AND BECK, C. S.: Present status of surgical procedures in chronic valvular disease of heart: final report of all surgical cases. Arch. Surg. *18:* 403, 1929.

24 ——, AND LEVINE, S. A.: Cardiotomy and valvulotomy for mitral stenosis. Experimental observations and clinical notes concerning operated case with recovery. Boston M. & S. J. *188:* 1023, 1923.

25 ——, ——, AND BECK, C. S.: Surgical treatment of mitral stenosis: experimental and clinical studies. Arch. Surg. *9:* 689, 1924.

26 DEXTER, L., GORLIN, R., LEWIS, B. M., SPIEGL, R. J., AND HAYNES, F. W.: Physiological evaluation of patients with mitral stenosis before and after mitral valvuloplasty. Proceedings 24th Scientific Session, Am. Heart Assoc., June 1951.

27 DOW, J. W., AND DEXTER, L.: Circulatory dynamics in atrial septal defect. J. Clin. Investigation *29:* 809, 1950.

28 DOYEN, E.: Chirurgie des malformations congenitales ou acquises du coeur. 26th Cong. de l'assoc. franc. de chir. Presse méd. *21:* 860, 1913.

29 DRAPER, A. J., BING, R. J., FRIEDLICH, A., HEIMBECKER, R., AND DAMMANN, J. F.: Physiological studies in pre and postoperative mitral stenosis. J. Clin. Investigation *29:* 809, 1950.

30 DURANT, T.: Cited by Bailey, C. P.: The surgical treatment of mitral stenosis. Dis. Chest. *15:* 377, 1949.

31 EDITORIAL: Surgical operation for mitral stenosis. Lancet. *1:* 461, 1902.

32 FERGUSON, F. C., KOBILAC, R. E., AND DIETRICK, J. E.: Varices of bronchial veins as source of hemoptysis in mitral stenosis. Am. Heart J. *28:* 445, 1944.

33 GLOVER, R. P., BAILEY, C. P., AND O'NEILL, T. J. E.: Surgery of stenotic valvular disease of the heart. J. A. M. A. *144:* 1049, 1950.

34 ——, O'NEILL, T. J. E., AND BAILEY, C. P.: Commissurotomy for mitral stenosis. Circulation *1:* 329, 1950.

[35] GORLIN, R., AND GORLIN, S. G.: Hydraulic formula for calculation of the area of the stenotic mitral valve, other cardiac valves, and central circulation shunts. Am. Heart J. *41:* 1, 1951.

[35] ——, HAYNES, F. W., GOODALE, W. T., SAWYER, C. G., DOW, J. W., AND DEXTER, L.: Studies of the circulatory dynamics in mitral stenosis. Am. Heart J. *41:* 30, 1951.

[37] GRANT, R. T.: After histories for ten years of a thousand men suffering from heart disease. Heart *6:* 275, 1933.

[38] HARKEN, D. E.: Personal communication, May 1951.

[39] ——, ELLIS, L. B., DEXTER, L., FARRAND, R. E., DICKSON, J. F., III: The responsibility of the physician in the selection of patients with mitral stenosis for surgical treatment. Circulation. In press.

[40] ——, ——, WARE, P. F., AND NORMAN, L. R.: The surgical treatment of mitral stenosis. I. Valvuloplasty. New England J. Med. *239:* 801, 1948.

[41] JAROTZKY, A.: Zur Frage der Operation im Innern des Herzens bei Stenosis mitralis. Zentralbl. f. Chir. *53:* 140, 1926.

[42] KLEBS, F.: Ueber operative verletzungender Herzklappen und deren Folgen. Prag. Med. Wchnschr. *1:* 29, 1876.

[43] LENÈGRE, J.: Personal communication, April 1951.

[44] LONGMIRE, W. P.: Personal communication from Dr. W. H. Muller, Jr. (and W. P. Longmire), May 1951.

[45] LUTEMBACHER, R.: De la sténose mitrale avec communication interauriculaire. Arch. mal. coeur *9:* 237, 1916.

[46] MACCALLUM, W. G., AND McCLURE, R. D.: On mechanical effects of experimental mitral stenosis and insufficiency. Bull. Johns Hopkins Hosp. *17:* 260, 1906.

[47] MURRAY, G.: Treatment of mitral valve stenosis by resection and replacement of valve under direct vision. Arch. Surg. *61:* 903, 1950.

[48] O'FARRELL, P. T.: The clinical diagnosis of congenital heart disease. Irish J. M. Sc. *153:* 608, 1938.

[49] PINCOFFS, M. C.: Discussion of "a venous shunt for mitral stenosis" (Bland-Sweet). Tr. Am. Clin. & Clim. Assoc. *48:* 77, 1948.

[50] POWERS, J. H.: The experimental production of mitral stenosis. Arch. Surg. *18:* 1945, 1929.

[51] ——: Surgical treatment of mitral stenosis: an experimental study. Arch. Surg. *25:* 554, 1932.

[52] PRIBRAM, B. O.: Die operative Behandlung der Mitralstenose. Arch. f. klin. Chir. *142:* 458, 1926.

[53] SCHEPELMANN, E.: Versuche zur Herzchirurgie. Arch. f. klin. Chir. *95:* 739, 1912.

[54] SMITHY, H. G.: An approach to the surgical treatment of chronic valvular disease of the heart. Read before the 16th Annual Assembly, Southeastern Surg. Congress, April 1948.

[55] ——, BOONE, J. A., AND STALLWORTH, J. M.: Surgical treatment of constrictive valvular disease of the heart. Surg. Gynec. & Obst. *90:* 175, 1950.

[56] ——, AND PARKER, E. F.: Experimental aortic valvulotomy: preliminary report. Surg. Gynec. & Obst. *84:* 625, 1947.

[57] SOUTTAR, H. S.: Surgical treatment of mitral stenosis. Brit. M. J. *2:* 603, 1925.

[58] SWAN, H.: Mitral stenosis, an experimental study of pulmonary-azygos venous anastomosis. Am. Heart J. *38:* 367, 1949.

[59] SWEET, R. H., AND BLAND, E. F.: Surgical relief of congestion in the pulmonary circulation in cases of severe mitral stenosis. Ann. Surg. *130:* 384, 1949.

[60] TUFFIER, T.: Etat actuel de la chirurgie intrathoracique. Tr. Internat. C. ng. Med. 1913, London, 1914; sect. 7, Surg. Part 2, p. 249, 1914.

The Management of Cardiac Patients in Relation to Surgery

By A. CARLTON ERNSTENE, M.D.

THE INTERNIST frequently is called upon by his surgical colleagues for an opinion concerning the risk of anesthesia and of a surgical procedure in a patient who has organic heart disease. A request of this kind carries with it a number of implied questions, among the most important of which are:

1. Does the cardiac abnormality increase the risk of the contemplated procedure?

2. Will the anesthesia and surgical operation increase the demands on the heart beyond the limits of the cardiac reserve and therefore precipitate congestive heart failure?

3. Does the cardiac condition require treatment before operation?

4. Is the prognosis of the heart condition so grave that surgery should be limited to an emergency or palliative procedure?

5. Is the heart disease of such a nature that it carries with it the liability of sudden death during anesthesia and surgical operation?

6. What bearing does the state of the heart have on the choice of the anesthetic agent?

7. What, if any, cardiovascular complications are to be anticipated during the operation and postoperative period?

The information necessary to answer these questions usually can be obtained from the clinical history and physical examination without resorting to more elaborate forms of investigation.

It still is quite commonly believed that during anesthesia and surgical operations the heart is subjected to a considerably increased demand for work, but there is no evidence that this is actually the case. The two greatest dangers to which a patient is exposed during an operation under general anesthesia are anoxia and shock. If these are avoided by proper anesthesia, minimizing of blood loss, and careful manipulation of tissues, even prolonged and extensive surgical procedures do not increase the load on the heart as much as does moderate physical exertion. Competent anesthesia is seldom attended by cyanosis or more than slight alterations in respiration, pulse rate, and blood pressure; and changes of this kind are encountered no more frequently in patients who have organic heart disease with a satisfactory myocardial and coronary reserve than in normal individuals. It may be taken as a general rule, therefore, that if anoxia and shock are avoided, patients with organic heart disease who have been able to carry on normal daily activities without experiencing symptoms of myocardial or coronary insufficiency can tolerate general anesthesia and surgery with no more hazard than a normal person.[1] There are a few exceptions to this rule, and these will be mentioned later. The presence of hypertension does not affect the validity of the general statement, provided that renal function has not been depressed to an important degree.

In estimating the risk of anesthesia and surgery in a patient who has organic heart disease, careful inquiry concerning dyspnea or substernal pain on exertion, paroxysmal nocturnal dyspnea, attacks of acute coronary failure, and former acute myocardial infarction is of much more importance than are the cardiac findings on physical examination. Certain findings, however, such as enlargement of the heart, murmurs indicative of valvular damage, gallop rhythm, and important disturbances of cardiac rhythm, may make it advisable to question the patient again in order to be certain that the questions have been understood and truthfully answered. The same consideration applies to the majority of electrocardiographic abnormalities. With few exceptions, an abnormal electrocardiogram in an individual who has had no symptoms of impaired myocardial or coronary reserve does not indicate added danger from anesthesia and surgery. As examples, bundle branch block does not of itself increase surgical mortality or postoperative morbidity,[2] and patients who have auricular fibrillation without congestive failure tolerate anesthesia and operation satisfactorily if the ventricular rate has been properly controlled by digitalis.

Occasionally a need for anesthesia and surgery arises in patients who are suffering from congestive heart failure. In such circumstances it is advisable that there be a period of preoperative treatment, the intensity and duration of which will be determined by the degree of failure and the urgency of the surgical condition. A surgical emergency, such as acute appendicitis or a perforated peptic ulcer, will not permit delay, and the risk of immediate operation must be accepted. If, in a situation of this kind, the patient has not been receiving digitalis, a suitable preparation of the drug should be administered by intravenous injection before the anesthesia is started. The dose usually employed is one-half or somewhat more of the amount estimated to be necessary for complete digitalization. After the operation additional intravenous or intramuscular injections of smaller amounts can be given at intervals of four hours or so until the process of digitalization is complete. One of the mercurial diuretics should be given by intramuscular injection at the same time as the initial dose of digitalis and subsequently each day until the preparation no longer causes diuresis or loss of weight.

When congestive heart failure is present and the surgical condition is of such nature that operation can be delayed safely for a few days or longer, digitalization should be accomplished by the oral route or, if nausea and vomiting are present, by the intramuscular injection of one of the preparations designed for this purpose. If auricular fibrillation is present, the ventricular rate furnishes the most helpful guide as to whether or not the maximum therapeutic effect of the drug has been obtained; sufficient digitalis is given to reduce the rate, in the absence of fever, severe anemia and thyrotoxicosis, to approximately 70 beats per minute. When normal rhythm is present, the heart rate is of no aid in estimating the degree of digitalization, and one must then prescribe the amount of the drug required by the average patient and be guided by the general clinical response. The sodium content of the diet should be strictly limited, and one of the mercurial diuretics should be administered. Surgery should be postponed, if at all possible, until all evidence of congestive failure has disappeared. If this is done, the patient can reasonably be expected to stand anesthesia and operation without difficulty, but if sufficient delay is impossible and adequate treatment cannot be carried out, surgery may be followed by a considerable increase in the degree of failure.

Regardless of the adequacy of preoperative treatment, patients who have had congestive failure before operation must be watched closely during the period after surgery. Postoperative complications, such as pulmonary embolism, atelectasis, pneumonia, and abdominal distention, are not well borne and may be responsible for a return of or an increase in the manifestations of decompensation. The mortality related to these complications is considerably greater in patients who have had congestive failure before operation than in normal individuals or in those who have organic heart disease with little or no impairment of myocardial reserve.

Digitalis also should be administered before operation to persons who do not have congestive failure but who have experienced dyspnea of cardiac origin on moderate exertion or paroxysmal nocturnal dyspnea. Although these patients usually tolerate anesthesia and operation satisfactorily without preoperative digitalization, the added strain of unforeseen postoperative complications may be sufficient to precipitate cardiac decompensation. The preparatory use of digitalis will improve the ability of the heart to withstand such an added strain so that postoperative mortality should not be significantly greater than in individuals who have a normal myocardial reserve. The amount of the drug given should be sufficient to accomplish theoretic digitalization, and the dosage schedule will be determined by the time available.

All patients who have auricular fibrillation or auricular flutter should be completely digitalized before operation whenever possible, even though there have been no symptoms of diminished myocardial reserve and regardless of the ventricular rate. As in the case of persons who have symptomatic myocardial insufficiency without congestive failure, these patients are seldom adversely affected by anesthesia and surgery. However, anoxia, hemorrhage or shock during operation, and such postoperative complications as pneumonia, atelectasis, thromboembolic accidents and abdominal distention are liable to cause an abnormally great increase in the ventricular rate in the absence of digitalis control. This in turn may result in the development of cardiac decompensation. Blumgart[3] demonstrated that a given amount of exercise causes a much greater rise in heart rate in individuals who have auricular fibrillation than it does in patients who have normal rhythm. After the administration of digitalis the response to exercise still remains greater than in persons with normal rhythm but the maximum ventricular rate attained is less than before the drug is used.

In the absence of symptoms of myocardial insufficiency, the presence of hypertension, enlargement of the heart, evidence of organic valvular disease, premature beats and electrocardiographic changes indicative of myocardial damage, preponderance of either ventricle or coronary artery disease are not to be considered indications for the preoperative use of digitalis. There is likewise no evidence that digitalis is of benefit in the preoperative care of elderly patients who have a normal myocardial reserve. Occasionally, however, an elderly individual is encountered who experiences dyspnea on exertion and yet presents no objective evidence of cardiac or pulmonary disease. The preoperative use of digitalis is warranted in such patients on the assumption that the dyspnea may be of cardiac origin even though no clear-cut proof is available.

In patients who have been able to carry on normal daily activities without experiencing symptoms of myocardial or coronary insufficiency, the fact that organic heart disease is present does not influence the decision as to the type of operation to be done. As in the case of persons with normal hearts, the procedure carried out should be the one required for the cure or correction of the surgical problem. The situation is different, however, when the heart condition is such that death from a cardiac cause must be anticipated within a period of two to four years at the most. All elective surgical procedures are then to be avoided. In patients who have had congestive heart failure, for example, the repair of abdominal or inguinal hernias should be postponed as long as the condition can be controlled reasonably well by mechanical means, and myomas of the uterus should be treated by radiation rather than by hysterectomy.

There are certain heart conditions which are liable to result in sudden death even under normal circumstances, and in patients who are in one of these states, the occurrence of even mild anoxia or shock during or after operation may directly precipitate the changes which abruptly terminate life. The conditions include angina pectoris, recent myocardial infarction, recent acute coronary failure, aortic stenosis, coronary ostial stenosis due to syphilitic aortitis, and high grade or complete auriculoventricular block complicated by the Adams-Stokes syndrome. Aortic stenosis and syphilitic aortitis may have caused no symptoms prior to the operation but the other conditions will have given rise to characteristic manifestations. In patients who have aortic stenosis or severe coronary disease, the most common cause of sudden death appears to be ventricular fibrillation which may or may not be preceded by a short paroxysm of ventricular tachycardia. Death from the Adams-Stokes syndrome is due, with rare exceptions, to ventricular asystole. In patients who have had angina pectoris, myocardial infarction, or acute coronary failure, the fall in blood pressure which accompanies surgical or postoperative shock may so reduce coronary blood flow that acute coronary failure or myocardial infarction results. Either of these, if not suddenly fatal, may be responsible for the rapid development of congestive heart failure. The risk of anesthesia and surgery in patients who have any of the forms of heart disease which are attended by the danger of sudden death must be recognized beforehand, and surgery should be carried out only when unavoidable. Everything possible must be done to prevent anoxia and a fall in blood pressure during the operation, and the surgical procedure employed must be the simplest one available. The risk must not be magnified beyond its true proportions, however, and patients must not be denied the benefit of surgery when an operation is necessary. Brumm and Willius[4] reported only 11 deaths (4.3 per cent) from cardiac causes in 257 patients with severe coronary disease who were subjected to required surgical procedures. Attacks of angina pectoris had been experienced by these patients for an average of 3.1 years, and 32 had healed infarcts at the time of operation. Death occurred from coronary thrombosis in 7, congestive heart failure in 2, and abruptly without apparent coronary occlusion in 2. In patients who have had myocardial infarction, operation should be postponed, if at all possible, for at least three months from the onset of the attack.

Mention has been made of the advisability of avoiding operation whenever possible in patients who have, or have had, congestive heart failure. This, of course, does not apply when myocardial failure is due in whole or in part to a condition which can be corrected by surgery. Cardiac decompensation occurs in approximately 4 per cent of all patients who have hyperthyroidism, the two most important factors responsible for its development being accompanying organic heart disease and uncontrolled auricular fibrillation. Correction of the thyrotoxicosis by radioactive iodine, or by subtotal thyroidectomy after thorough preoperative preparation, usually restores myocardial reserve to a normal or nearly normal level. Reversion to sinus rhythm occurs spontaneously in approximately one-third of those patients in whom auricular fibrillation was present, and normal rhythm can be re-established in about one-half of the remainder by the administration of quinidine. Arteriovenous aneurysm, patent ductus arteriosus and chronic constrictive pericarditis also may be responsible for the development of congestive heart failure. Treatment by the measures ordinarily employed for cardiac decompensation is of limited value but surgical correction of the causative condition usually results in complete disappearance of the manifestations of failure.

Because skillfully administered inhalation anesthesia does not increase the work of the heart, the presence of organic heart disease is only occasionally of more than secondary importance in determining the choice of the anesthetic agent. The type of operation and the general condition of the patient usually are the deciding factors. Nitrous oxide–oxygen and ethylene–oxygen, supplemented by ether if necessary, are well tolerated by patients with organic heart disease when strict precautions are taken to avoid anoxia. Sodium Pentothal by intravenous injection may be used for minor procedures and for operations which do not require relaxation of the abdominal muscles if at the same time 100 per cent oxygen is administered by inhalation. Cyclopropane should not be used because of the possibility of inducing important ventricular arrhythmias. In this connection it should be emphasized that the administration of epinephrine during cyclopropane anesthesia is an extremely hazardous procedure. Cyclopropane sensitizes the heart to epinephrine so that the latter drug readily causes ventricular tachycardia and ventricular fibrillation.[5]

In the presence of one of the forms of heart disease which is likely to cause sudden death, local anesthesia should be employed if possible. The same cardiac conditions contraindicate the use of spinal anesthesia whenever the required operation can be performed under some other agent. A pronounced drop in arterial blood pressure due to spinal anesthesia may reduce coronary blood flow to such a degree that fatal cardiac arrhythmias, acute coronary failure or myocardial infarction result. The administration of Neosynephrine by subcutaneous or intramuscular injection greatly reduces the incidence of dangerous hypotension, and therefore diminishes the risk when spinal anesthesia must be used.[6] Pituitrin should not be employed to combat the hypotensive effects of spinal anesthesia in patients with organic heart disease because of its constrictive action on the coronary arteries.

Important cardiovascular complications are uncommon during operations skillfully performed under competent anesthesia. Disturbances of cardiac rhythm occur with considerable frequency but only occasionally are they of such a nature as to be of clinical significance. Kurtz, Bennett and Shapiro[7] observed abnormalities in the electrocardiograms of nearly 80 per cent of 109 patients subjected to surgery, the incidence of changes being higher in persons with abnormal hearts than in those without heart disease. The most common alterations consisted of sinus arrhythmia, premature beats and downward displacement of the pacemaker. More important arrhythmias occurred in only seven instances.

In a recent study of electrocardiographic changes during cyclopropane-ether anesthesia, Johnstone[13] reported the frequent occurrence of sinus bradycardia and A-V nodal rhythm. The changes apparently were due to reflex vagal inhibition of the heart secondary to stimulation of nerve endings in the air passages by the anesthetic agent. In one patient, sinus bradycardia progressed to transient complete cardiac arrest. Atropine prevented extreme sinus bradycardia but, in doses of less than 1.2 mg., did not affect the incidence of A-V nodal rhythm. It was observed, however, that if carbon dioxide was allowed to accumulate in the anesthesia circuit, atropine might induce ventricular tachycardia or frequent ventricular premature beats. Attention also was directed to the fact that the simultaneous administration of atropine and prostigmine may result in the development of ventricular fibrillation. Prostigmine has been employed as an antidote for overdosage with curare, and in order to avoid its use Johnstone recommends that only a single dose of curare be given to any patient. Muscular relaxation should be maintained subsequently by anesthetic agents and not by the administration of more curare.

Anoxia, shock and a considerable drop in blood pressure during anesthesia and surgery may be responsible for the development of premature beats even in patients who have perfectly normal hearts. When anoxia is the cause, the arrhythmia frequently can be abolished promptly by increasing the oxygen content of the anesthetic mixture. If the premature beats are of ventricular origin and occur with increasing frequency in spite of added amounts of oxygen, they may be eliminated by the intravenous administration of procaine amide hydrochloride (Pronestyl) in doses of 100 to 500 mg. The same preparation is of value in terminating ventricular tachycardia during anesthesia. The drug may be useful also in the treatment of supraventricular tachycardia. Tachycardia of the latter type, as well as that of ventricular origin, often can be brought to an end by the intravenous injection of procaine hydrochloride in doses of 30 to 70 mg.[8]

The two most serious cardiac complications of inhalation anesthesia are standstill of the heart and ventricular fibrillation. Both conditions cause sudden disappearance of arterial pulsations and audible heart beats, and the electrocardiogram or direct inspection of the heart therefore is necessary to distinguish one from the other. Cardiac arrest and ventricular fibrillation are rare occurrences but either may develop without warning during any type of surgical procedure and in the entire absence of organic heart disease. Both can be treated successfully if the diagnosis is made promptly and treatment started within three to five minutes. Because accurate recognition is of such fundamental importance, the time may well come when an inexpensive oscilloscope will be a part of every anesthetist's armamentarium. There must also be a plan of action to be followed whenever such an emergency arises. The procedure to be followed is the one recommended by Beck.[9] Once the diagnosis is made, the heart should be exposed without delay. The practice of intracardiac injection of epinephrine through the chest wall should be discouraged because it involves loss of time and may be responsible for the development of ventricular fibrillation in a heart in standstill. Having exposed the heart, the surgeon immediately begins cardiac massage, usually at a rate of approximately 40 contractions per minute, and only after this has been carried on for a few minutes does he stop momentarily to ascertain whether the condition is one of standstill or ventricular fibrillation. In the event of standstill, massage is resumed and is continued until spontaneous cardiac contractions appear. The first beats may be very feeble, and if they do not increase in strength, 1 cc. of 1:1000 epinephrine is injected into the chamber of the right auricle or ventricle. This is the only situation in which epinephrine should be employed in cardiac resuscitation. When ventricular fibrillation is present, 5 per cent procaine is applied to the surface of the heart, and cardiac massage is continued without interruption. If the arrhythmia persists, 5 cc. of a 2 per cent procaine solution are next injected into the right auricle or right ventricle. Massage is continued, and if the disturbance is not terminated, electric shock is next employed. Alternating current of 1 to 1.5 amperes is applied to the heart for a fraction of a second through special electrodes.

Postoperative cardiac complications are not common and are seldom responsible for death of the patient. The greatest incidence is encountered in individuals who have severe coronary artery disease.[10, 11] In these patients, death may be due to acute myocardial infarction, congestive heart failure or the sudden development of ventricular fibrillation. Master and his associates[12] found that of 625 instances of coronary occlusion, 35 (5.6 per cent) occurred following some surgical procedure.

Auricular fibrillation occurs as a relatively unimportant postoperative complication in approximately 10 per cent of all patients subjected to thyroidectomy for hyperthyroidism. The arrhythmia generally begins within the first two or three days after operation and usually lasts for less than 48 hours. It seldom requires special treatment, although it seems advisable to begin gradual digitalization at its onset. One of the serious complications to which patients with mitral stenosis and auricular fibrillation are subject is an embolic accident due to dislodgment of a portion of a mural thrombus in the auricular appendages. A development of this kind, however, is no more likely to occur during surgical operations or the postoperative period than at other times.

There is one feature of the postoperative management of patients who have organic heart disease which deserves emphasis. This has to do with the administration of fluids by intravenous injection. All preparations which contain sodium, including whole blood and plasma, should be avoided unless their use is specifically indicated. When fluids must be given, the solution employed should consist only of 5 per cent glucose in distilled water whenever possible. In the presence of organic heart disease the administration of large amounts of sodium-containing fluids may be directly responsible for the appearance of pulmonary edema and other features of congestive heart failure even though there may have been no symptoms of myocardial insufficiency before operation. The danger is, of course, particularly great in patients who have congestive failure before operation even though all manifestations of decompensation have been controlled satisfactorily by treatment before surgery is undertaken. Occurrences of this kind probably have not been too uncommon in the past and undoubtedly have been a factor in furthering the erroneous belief that patients who have organic heart disease do not tolerate anesthesia and surgical operations satisfactorily.

The occurrences of pneumonia, atelectasis, thromboembolic accidents, and abdominal distention during the postoperative period constitute especially great dangers for patients who have organic heart disease and may be responsible for the initial development or return of congestive heart failure. The antibiotic drugs, early ambulation, prompt use of anticoagulants on the first appearance of evidence of phlebothrombosis, and continuous gastric suction have greatly reduced the incidence of these complications and have therefore improved the outlook of cardiac patients who require surgery.

Summary

Skillful anesthesia and surgical operations do not significantly increase the demands upon the heart for work. Patients who have organic heart disease but who have been able to carry on normal daily activities without symptoms referable to the heart tolerate anesthesia and operation without difficulty provided that anoxia, hemorrhage and shock are avoided. Hypertension, cardiac enlargement, valvular disease other than advanced aortic stenosis, and electrocardiographic abnormalities, per se, do not increase surgical mortality or postoperative morbidity. When symptomatic myocardial insufficiency or evidence of congestive heart failure is present, a period of preoperative treatment with rest, digitalis, sodium restriction and mercurial diuretics is advisable. Treatment should be as thorough as possible during the interval in which the operation can be safely delayed. With adequate management, patients who have had myocardial failure can be expected to tolerate anesthesia and surgery satisfactorily. Postoperative complications, such as pneumonia, atelectasis, thromboembolic accidents and abdominal distention, are not well borne, however, and may be responsible for a return of cardiac decompensation.

Patients who have auricular fibrillation or auricular flutter should be digitalized before operation even though there have been no symptoms of impaired myocardial reserve and regardless of the ventricular rate.

Surgery should be avoided if possible in persons who have severe coronary disease, aortic stenosis, coronary ostial stenosis due to syphilitic aortitis, and high grade or complete auriculoventricular block complicated by the Stokes-Adams syndrome. Spinal anesthesia should not be employed in the presence of these conditions.

The decision as to the exact type of operation to be performed is seldom influenced by the existence of organic heart disease.

The presence of organic heart disease is only occasionally of more than secondary importance in determining the choice of the anesthetic agent to be given by inhalation. Cyclopropane, however, should not be used.

Although unimportant disturbances of cardiac rhythm occur frequently during anesthesia and operation, serious complications such as ventricular tachycardia, standstill of the heart and ventricular fibrillation are uncommon. The treatment of these conditions has been discussed.

Postoperative cardiac complications are not common and are seldom responsible for death of the patient. The greatest incidence occurs in patients who have severe coronary artery disease.

The intravenous administration of fluids which contain sodium should be avoided during operation and the postoperative period unless their use is specifically indicated.

ACKNOWLEDGMENT

This work is from the Cleveland Clinic and the Frank E. Bunts Educational Institute, Cleveland, Ohio.

REFERENCES

[1] MARVIN, H. M.: The heart during anesthesia and operative procedures. New England J. Med. *199:* 547, 1928.

[2] PFEIFFER, P. H., AND LADUE, J. S.: Major surgical operations in the presence of bundle branch block. Am. J. M. Sc. *217:* 369, 1949.

[3] BLUMGART, H. L.: The reaction to exercise of the heart affected by auricular fibrillation. Heart *11:* 49, 1924.

[4] BRUMM, H. J., AND WILLIUS, F. A.: The surgical risk in patients with coronary disease. J. A. M. A. *112:* 2377, 1939.

[5] MEEK, W. J.: Cardiac automaticity and response to blood pressure raising agents during inhalation anesthesia. Physiol. Rev. *21:* 324, 1941.

[6] BELLINKOFF, S.: The choice of anesthesia in cardiac disease. Anesthesiology *7:* 268, 1946.

[7] KURTZ, C. M., BENNETT, J. H., AND SHAPIRO, H. H.: Electrocardiographic studies during surgical anesthesia. J. A. M. A. *106:* 434, 1936.

[8] BURSTEIN, C.: Treatment of acute arrhythmias during anesthesia by intravenous procaine. Anesthesiology *7:* 113, 1946.

[9] BECK, C. S.: Resuscitation for cardiac standstill and ventricular fibrillation occurring during operation. Am. J. Surg. *54:* 273, 1941.

[10] BUTLER, S., FEENEY, N., AND LEVINE, S. A.: The patient with heart disease as a surgical risk. J. A. M. A. *95:* 85, 1930.

[11] MORRISON, D. R.: Risk of surgery in heart disease. Surgery *23:* 561, 1948.

[12] MASTER, A. M., DACK, S., AND JAFFE, H. L.: Postoperative coronary artery occlusion. J. A. M. A. *110:* 1415, 1938.

[13] JOHNSTONE, M.: General anaesthesia and cardiac inhibition. Brit. Heart J. *13:* 4, 1951.

Emotion and the Circulation

By MARK D. ALTSCHULE, M.D.

ACCEPTANCE of the Platonic doctrine that all bodily ills proceed from the spirit led medical authors of antiquity, the Middle Ages and the Renaissance to ascribe cardiac diseases to emotional disorders almost exclusively. Postmortem studies, impressively collected by various authors, notably Zimmerman,[1] appeared to confirm this general idea and to support such concepts as "dying of a broken heart," where cardiac rupture was found in grief, or "hardness of heart," in which pericarditis was found in individuals notorious for cruelty. In the early nineteenth century, Corvisart and his followers, Burns, Testa and Kreysing, likewise believed emotion to be the most important cause of heart disease. The cause of cardiac and aortic dilatations was confidently stated to be the driving inward of the bodily humors during psychic stress. Sudden development of dropsy, cardiac hypertrophy and aortic aneurysms immediately following a single severe emotional upset was often described. Corvisart and Testa stated that heart disease increased markedly during and after the French Revolution and attributed this phenomenon to the disorder of the times. Bertin, a decade later, held that seeming increases in cardiac disease were due only to its being recognized more certainly. This controversy of over a century ago sounds familiar in the present. In spite of increase of knowledge of pathologic anatomy in the nineteenth century, etiologies of cardiovascular diseases remained obscure. The tendency to ascribe conditions of unknown etiology to emotional disturbances persisted, as exemplified by one authority of the 1870's, who stated with assurance "It is not surprising that in the present day, when the worry of life and strain on the feelings in all ways are so vastly intensified, that there should be strong evidence to show the increase of cardiac affections"; Balfour expressed similar ideas 25 years later and today some cardiovascular diseases still are considered to be due to psychic disorder.

The problem that plagues the cardiologist arises from the fact that he sees evidence daily on the influence of emotion on the circulation but has at hand no extensive body of physiologic data that might illuminate his clinical observations. For the most part, the psychosomatic studies of the circulation merely emphasize what the competent internist appreciates, namely, that emotion may cause cardiovascular symptoms. The present discussion will analyze available physiologic studies and will attempt to relate them to clinical phenomena. Reference will be made only to the heart and peripheral blood vessels; consideration of renal and gastrointestinal circulation will be omitted.

Peripheral Vascular System

Physicians of antiquity believed that specific emotions caused specific changes in the pulse; this belief has persisted, in various forms, during the past 25 centuries. For instance, early in the present century, Wundt, in his *Gefuhlstheorie*, classified feelings rigidly in three pairs, i.e., pleasure-pain, tension-relaxation, and excitation-calm, and his followers claimed to have observed specific changes in the pulse wave corresponding with each. This work, reviewed by Leshke[2] in 1914, formed a seemingly convincing body of evidence which now is regarded as invalid. Recent work on specificity in peripheral vascular reactions to emotion[3] evokes doubt because of skepticism regarding the authors' ability to characterize exactly the feelings experienced by their subjects during short experiments and because of the absence of suitable control periods.

Many physiologic studies of general effects of psychic factors on peripheral circulation are available.[4] Cutaneous vasoconstriction in the hands and feet during emotion has been amply demonstrated; this change manifests itself by cooling of the parts and, because of stasis, excessive deoxygenation of the capillary blood. In ordinary circumstances, changes in the hands are due both to arteriolar and venular constriction, whereas those in the forearm are largely venular in origin; on the arterial side only the terminal cutaneous arteries, and not the radial, metacarpal and digital arteries, usually are involved. In extremely severe emotion, however, spasm of the radial artery may be detected. As a consequence of spasm of arterioles and venules, changes in cutaneous capillaries occur; these are visible on microscopic examination of the vessels of the fingernail folds. All the changes described are minimized by vasodilating agents such as alcohol, carbon dioxide or warmth.

The immediate vasoconstriction of emotion is effected via the sympathetic nervous system and a sympathectomized extremity does not show it. The hypothalamus contains centers governing generalized vasoconstriction and vasodilatation but the occurrence in emotional states of vasomotor changes limited commonly to the acral areas raises the possibility that the impulses arise in the cortex. On the other hand, it is possible that vasomotor changes in general are most marked in the acral regions so that weak discharges from the hypothalamic centers cause changes which are detectable only in the extremities. At any rate, the importance of cortical impulses in vasomotor phenomena is now recognized; this will be discussed below, in relation to hypertension.

Although most studies of peripheral flow emphasize unpleasant emotions in causing the changes observed, there are data which show that strong pleasurable emotions may give rise to identical peripheral vascular phenomena.[5] The thesis that subjects who show marked vasomotor changes with pleasurable emotions are expressing subconscious guilt consequent to experiencing such feelings is not supported by psychologic studies. In addition, as Lombard showed a century ago, and others have corroborated since,[6] vasoconstriction in the extremities occurs also during concentration not obviously emotionally colored.

Peripheral vasomotor phenomena of emotion do not parallel regularly the facial expression of emotion and even less so the verbal description of it. Whether conscious or unconscious feelings are the more important is unknown; however, emotional vasoconstriction disappears during sleep, when, according to psychoanalytic thinking, unconscious emotions are at their height.

Patients with persistent and marked emotional vasoconstriction exhibit coldness of the extremities and are intolerant to cold temperatures. Confusion may arise with the symptoms of hypothyroidism or anemia so that patients may needlessly receive thyroid or antianemic medications.

The vasoconstrictor effects of emotion may aggravate manifestations of such peripheral vascular diseases as arteriosclerosis, thromboangiitis obliterans, post-traumatic causalgia and Raynaud's disease.

In addition, men with a previous history of excessive vasomotor reaction to emotion are markedly susceptible to frost-bite and trench foot.[7, 8] Rheumatoid arthritis of the hands and feet is also demonstrably influenced by emotions and excessive vasoconstriction in this disease actually has been demonstrated.[9]

Fragmentary observations[10] suggest that subjects with unstable peripheral vascular systems develop conditioned reflexes involving this system more easily than do others; this may suggest a possible mechanism whereby the peripheral vascular system becomes the one which expresses emotion in some individuals. In addition, emotionally unstable individuals exhibit excessive acral vasoconstriction as a consequence of concentration itself,[6] which suggests that vasomotor as well as cerebral emotional mechanisms may be abnormal.

Physiologic phenomena underlying blushing and blanching of the face and neck have not been studied; here is a promising field for observation on specificity of emotional responses, for blanching with fear and blushing with embarrassment are well known. On the other hand, various feelings may cause either pallor or flushing in different individuals or in the same individuals at different times. The belief that easy blushing is evidence of a marked paranoid personality has no support in extensive observation, and is a conclusion based on an a priori interpretation of the symptom. Vasodilatation consequent to fever, external heat, imbibing of alcohol, or emotional upset is known to be followed by urticaria in some individuals.[11] Acetylcholine is released locally during vasodilatation and it is well known that acetylcholine is a whealing agent. Whether it acts as such, or through the liberation of histamine, is not established, however. Development of hives under these circumstances in some individuals and not in others is not understood.

Cardiac Rate

Marked changes in heart rate occur in relation to emotion. Poor correlation between changes in pulse rate and the facial or verbal expression of emotion is regularly found.[12] Variation in rate from minute to minute may be marked.[12] As a rule the rate is accelerated in emotional reactions but at times it may be abnormally slow. In some instances the sinus bradycardia is part of a syncopal reaction, while in others the bradycardia is not the precursor of any such reaction. The cause of the rapid and marked variation in rate is not known, although at times it may be due to sinus arrhythmia correlated with hyperventilation.

Changes in pulse rate during strong emotion are of the same magnitude in normal and in neurotic subjects. Neurotic subjects, however, experience more severe emotional reactions than normal subjects during mild stresses. The neurotic may, moreover, be more aware of emotional tachycardia than the non-neurotic subject. The pulse rate in exercise in neurotic subjects will be discussed below, in relation to neurocirculatory asthenia.

The relation of emotional tachycardia to conscious appreciation of emotions has not been defined. Emotional tachycardia subsides during sleep, a fact used in differentiating anxiety from thyrotoxicosis. On the other hand, during sleep a noise, insufficient to awaken the sleeper or make him exhibit overt evidence of startle, may increase the pulse rate by a third.[12] This phenomenon appears to vary with the depth of unconsciousness.

It is generally presumed that tachycardia of emotion is related to sympathetic hyperactivity, or production of excess epinephrine. However, norepinephrine, which does not increase pulse rate but merely raises the blood pressure, is probably liberated from the adrenal medulla together with epinephrine. An additional complication arises from the fact that acetylcholine in small amount causes tachycardia and in larger amount slows the pulse. It is known also that the brain contains areas which cause tachycardia when stimulated. It is evident that the precise cause of emotional tachycardia is not known.

Rapid heart rates in neurosis may lead to mistaken diagnoses of heart disease or thyrotoxicosis; neurotic patients who complain of tachycardia may be given antithyroid drugs or digitalis and may become disabled owing to bad advice regarding activity. It should be noted that palpitation in neurosis need not signify occurrence of a rapid heart rate; palpitation may be experienced with normal or slow heart rates if sudden rises in blood pressure occur, if the rhythm is irregular, or, on occasion, with no change in the circulatory mechanisms.

Cardiac Rhythm

Routine examination of neurotic subjects may not reveal the occurrence of any arrhythmia other than sinus arrhythmia, but every cardiologist has seen occasional instances in which auricular flutter, fibrillation or tachycardia, frequent auricular, nodal or ventricular premature beats, the Wolff-Parkinson-White syndrome, or minor degrees of heart block appear recurrently in emotionally unstable individuals without heart disease. At times the arrhythmia apparently develops in relation to some unusual emotional stress, but on other occasions similar stresses do not cause it; conversely, the arrhythmia may appear in the absence of overt emotional upset. The same fact holds in patients with established diagnoses of organic heart disease; partial heart block may increase in degree, or premature beats may become more numerous during emotional upset. The arrhythmias seen in relation to emotion are usually those produced by hyperactivity of the vagus nerve, i.e., arrhythmias involving the S-A node, the auricles and the A-V node; in the case of ventricular premature beats the effect of circulating epinephrine, or of sympathetic stimulation must be considered.

Electrocardiogram

Papers claiming that abnormalities of QRS complex or of T waves indicative of altered myocardial function occur in neuroses or are produced in normal subjects by emotion are unconvincing; changes shown appear to be due to variations in cardiac rate and in position of the heart. Examination made here of several hundred electrocardiograms in instances of emotional disorder corroborates the findings of others who showed no deviation from the normal.

Cardiac Output and Work: Circulation Time

That measurement of cardiac output in tense or frightened subjects yields values that are high relative to the basal has long been known to physiologists. The earlier work of Grollman[13] and the more recent studies of Stead and co-workers[14] and Hickam and associates,[15] all employing accurate methods, showed that emotion may increase cardiac output by two-thirds, and occasionally more; the cardiac output may vary markedly from minute to minute. These observations showed no relation between type of emotion and change in cardiac output. Hickam and co-workers[15] and Wolff and Wolff,[16] using the ballistocardiograph, found greater increases in cardiac output in many patients during emotional stresses; the latter authors claimed that some types of emotion caused decreases in the output of the heart. The ballistocardiograph is not accurate when the pulse rate changes markedly and rapidly. Discrepancies between the work of Wolff and Wolff[16] and that of other authors may be due to the method used; however, the observations of Hickam and associates,[15] who used the same method, do not support the concept of relation between type of emotion and circulatory change. Rises in cardiac output owing to emotion are greater than increases in oxygen consumption which occur at the same time; the cardiovascular changes resemble those which follow injection of small amounts of epinephrine.[15] Cardiac work is proportionately increased.

Circulation time is usually accelerated in emotional tension although marked emotionally-induced venoconstriction in the forearm may cause some slowing in the observed time and so give no true indication of the increase in cardiac output.

Change in cardiac output during anxiety in patients with heart disease but without failure are similar to those in normal subjects[15, 17]; in congestive failure, however, little or no increase in cardiac output (and work) occurs during anxiety although the pulse rate rises. The increase in metabolism induced by emotion in these circumstances results in further deoxygenation of capillary blood and exacerbation of the anoxia already present.

Stevenson and his co-workers[17] studied the effects of exercise on cardiac output in anxiety and found the rise to reach higher absolute values and also in some instances to be greater in amount than when the subjects exercised while relaxed. Makinson[18] found the increase to be normal but more prolonged in neurosis. However, the use of a method of low accuracy makes acceptance of these data only tentative. Nevertheless a metabolic effect of emotion, i.e., failure to oxidize carbohydrate completely, as described below, suggests that the cost of work is higher during stress and therefore the circulatory response in exercise should be greater than in normal circumstances.

Increases in resting cardiac output by about half owing to anxiety is not significant in causing emotional dyspnea during exertion except when the effort attempted is maximal; the maximal possible cardiac output is not approached during moderate physical activity and the patient does not need the cardiac reserve lost as a result of the increase in resting cardiac output occasioned by emotion. In patients with serious organic heart disease but no failure, the increases in cardiac output during strong emotion, may, if long continued, act in a manner like that of thyrotoxicosis, anemia, fever and other conditions which strain the heart and precipitate decompensation.

Cardiac Discomfort: Sudden Death

A variety of sensations seemingly localized about the heart occur during emotional reactions. The clutching discomfort occasioned by fear is well known; it differs from angina pectoris, according to those who have experienced both. The heavy sensation associated with sadness is also commonly experienced. The mechanism of these sensations is completely unknown.

Another type of discomfort, commonly seen in neurosis and more particularly in neurocirculatory asthenia, is the typical persistent, sticking pain close to the left breast. Its occurrence does not depend on changes in cardiac rate or rhythm, although in occasional patients it occurs only with premature beats or with palpitation. The mechanism of its production and the pathways of its transmission are not known. Commonly it is associated with persistent tenderness over the left chest although each of the two symptoms may occur without the other. Anxiety pain is occasionally confused with angina pectoris, leading to induction of a needless state of invalidism in the patient; this occurrence is a reflection on the physician who makes the error, for anxiety pain and anginal pain have only the most superficial resemblance. The confusion between anxiety pain and angina pectoris vitiates all of Dunbar's work[19] on the latter disorder.

Attacks of true angina pectoris may be precipitated by "disturbance of the mind," in the words of Herberden. In the presence of coronary arterial insufficiency, increases in cardiac work owing to emotion may cause anginal pain or may cause exertion more readily to induce it. John Hunter, whose clinical history and postmortem findings contributed to the modern theory of angina pectoris, often stated, "My life is at the mercy of any scoundrel who chooses to put me in a passion." Hunter's death occurred during a dispute with the Governors of St. George's Hospital regarding the exclusion of students whom he considered to be victims of a prejudice against the Scotch. The pain of angina pectoris occurs when the work of the heart is increased to a degree which cannot be paralleled by increased flow through diseased coronary arteries; the importance ascribed by Wolff and Wolff[16] to their findings of a lowered cardiac output in one patient during one attack of angina induced by emotion may be criticized in view of the fragmentary data, obtained by a method of low accuracy.

Another possible mechanism for the precipitation of anginal pain during emotional stress has not been studied adequately. That cooling of the skin of the hands favors the occurrence of anginal attacks in patients with the syndrome has been established[20, 21]; the fact that strong emotion usually causes cooling of the skin over the acral areas may therefore be significant.

Discussion of mechanisms for producing anginal attacks applies also to myocardial infarction. Sudden death during emotional strain has been recognized for at least 25 centuries as a common occurrence in the middle-aged or elderly. Although ventricular fibrillation may account for some, in many such instances myocardial infarction is the cause for this accident; it must not be concluded, however, that strong emotion is the sole or the most important cause of myocardial infarction. That strong pleasurable emotions may be as dangerous in causing sudden death as grief, rage or despair is important in relation to advising patients regarding their daily activities. Benjamin Rush described how ". . . the door-keeper of Congress, an aged man, died suddenly, immediately after hearing of the capture of Lord Cornwallis's army. His death was universally ascribed to a violent emotion of political joy. This species of joy appears to be one of the strongest emotions that can agitate the human mind."

Syncope

A fundamental phenomenon in syncope is strong vagal discharge causing marked sinus bradycardia; occasionally minor degrees of heart block and ventricular escape may occur. Total peripheral resistance decreases markedly and blood pressure falls[22]; there is also evidence of generalized loss of venous tone and, to judge from the cutaneous vasoconstriction which develops,[23] of pooling of blood in the viscera. The cutaneous vasoconstriction, manifested by disappearance of visible capillaries in the fingernail fold and by smallness of the superficial veins of the arm, may result from a sympathetic discharge elicited by the falling blood pressure. Cardiac output measured with the patient recumbent is normal,[22] but in the upright position it is markedly decreased.[23] In animals stimulation of areas in the frontal lobes causes hypotension and bradycardia; the relation of these findings to emotional syncope may be important.

Tendencies to recurrent fainting in neurotic patients may be ameliorated by the drugs effective against increased vagal tone, i.e., atropine, ephedrine and the like.

Hypertension

Much has been written on the importance of emotion in hypertension and opinions vary. Most cardiologists believe that psychic influences are among those which most strongly influence the course of the disease; on the other hand, some internists and most psychiatrists feel that emotional factors actually cause essential hypertension. The first of these opinions is well established but the second is not securely founded in observation. The present discussion will not attempt to resolve this issue but only to point out certain factors that must be borne in mind in considering it. Hypertension may cause only mild symptoms and accordingly introverted patients are most aware of these minor complaints; high incidence of neurosis in patients with complaints of hypertension therefore results. Also, since emotional upset does aggravate hypertension, the incidence of neurosis is high in patients with early or moderate hypertension. In addition, stresses of various types cause more marked and more persistent increases in blood pressure in neurotic than in normal subjects. Definition of physiologic mechanisms responsible for exacerbation of hypertension is difficult in the present state of knowledge, a fact that has not deterred many authors from doing so. There are observations which show that anxiety in normal or neurotic subjects is accompanied by decreased peripheral resistance; the diastolic blood pressure is elevated only occasionally and remains unchanged or falls for the most part. The systolic pressure rises parallel with increases in cardiac output.[14-17] These changes resemble effects of injection of small amounts of epinephrine. However, there is good evidence that shows that in essential hypertension the peripheral resistance is increased, both systolic and diastolic pressures rising, while the cardiac output remains normal. It is evident that the cardiovascular physiology of essential hypertension differs from that of anxiety. Nevertheless it is true that anxiety further elevates systolic pressure in hypertensive subjects and increases cardiac work greatly. The fact that norepinephrine is also liberated during stimulation of the adrenal medulla is also important. It acts entirely on peripheral blood vessels, increasing peripheral resistance and not influencing cardiac output directly, thereby producing changes resembling those of essential hypertension. To assume that one adrenal medullary hormone alone, epinephrine, is liberated during stress in normotensive subjects while the other, norepinephrine, is liberated alone in hypertensive subjects is not reasonable; however, work should be done to ascertain whether stress of short duration results largely in epinephrine effects, while stress of long duration causes predominately norepinephrine effects, as work of Bulbring and Burns[24] suggests may be possible.

The cold-pressor test in normotensive patients with anxiety causes rises in blood pressure which at most are only slightly greater than normal[25] and are much smaller than those found in hypertensive patients or some of their normotensive siblings. This finding again suggests that anxiety is not fundamental to essential hypertension.

Another humoral mechanism has been invoked to explain how anxiety may cause lasting hypertension. Decrease in renal blood flow, consequent to renal vasoconstriction, may occur in emotional stress; it has been suggested that renal ischemia so induced may give rise to elaboration of renin, and so cause elevation of both systolic and diastolic pressures without increasing cardiac output. Against this hypothesis is the fact that renin is not found in the blood in essential hypertension. In addition, not all patients with essential hypertension exhibit the changes in renal vascular dynamics required by this concept.

Excellent work in animals and more recently in man[26] has extended knowledge bearing on nervous pathways which carry vasoconstrictor impulses from the brain. Existence of vasoconstrictor centers in the hypothalamus has long been known; recently it has been shown that stimulation of the frontal cortex, especially that of its posterior orbital surface, elevates blood pressure. The location of this area in the general region in which is situated cortical representation of visceral changes and of somatic movements associated with expression of emotion is highly significant.

Some patients with essential hypertension exhibit significant changes in blood pressure in relation to variations in the intake of salt. The fact that a tendency toward salt retention may possibly exist during emotional stress, as discussed below, makes it necessary to consider this mechanism as possibly involved in relations between emotion and hypertension in some patients.

In spite of uncertainties regarding the manner in which emotion exacerbates hypertension, clinical observations nevertheless put the relationship between the two on a sound basis; observation thus far, however, lends no support to the concept that emotion causes essential hypertension. Statements that certain types of personality or emotional conflict are the cause of the disorder are ill-founded and should be received with skepticism.

Neurocirculatory Asthenia

The importance of neurocirculatory asthenia has been rediscovered during every war in the course of the last century; there is no evidence that it is increasing in frequency. Its relation to neurosis is indicated not only by the nature of its symptoms, but also by the fact that the physiologic changes induced by exercise in patients with various types of neurosis are similar to those considered characteristic of neurocirculatory asthenia. A physiologic difference between these two groups of patients lies in the fact that on the average changes are greater in neurocirculatory asthenia; however, there is much overlapping of the two groups.[27]

In addition to pain and precordial tenderness discussed above, symptoms pertinent to the present discussion consist in diminution in tolerance to exercise owing to abnormally severe palpitation, dyspnea, or fatigue.

In emotionally disturbed subjects, exercise causes a greater rise in pulse rate than in the same subject when not upset, or in normal subjects; the pulse rate falls slowly after the exercise. The mechanism underlying this phenomenon is not known; the concept held in some quarters that hyperventilation is the cause of the tachycardia is not securely founded. The severity of the palpitation, due both to the markedly abnormal pulse rate and also to the patients' increased awareness of symptoms, results in disinclination toward exercise. If tachycardia is very marked during exercise in a neurotic subject it is possible that some impairment of circulatory function might develop owing to lessened filling of the heart due to shortening of diastole.

Otherwise tachycardia is important only because of discomfort it may cause.

To consider neurocirculatory asthenia solely as a state in which the flesh is willing but the spirit weak is an error, for when patients with neurocirculatory asthenia, or indeed with neurosis, exercise, evidence of a metabolic disorder becomes evident[27, 28]; minor degrees of this disorder may be apparent at rest also. The resting blood lactate level may be slightly elevated in some, but during exercise it rises regularly to a higher level and remains elevated longer than in normal subjects doing the same work. Oxygen consumption during strenuous work is not increased as much as in normal subjects and consequently there is a large and prolonged oxygen debt. Associated with excessive and prolonged rises in blood lactate in exercise there are corresponding increases in respiration, so that the carbon dioxide content of expired air falls and carbon dioxide may be washed out of the blood; during work the respiratory rate and minute volume increase more than in normal subjects and remain elevated for an abnormally long period after the end of exertion.

Mechanisms responsible for this metabolic phenomenon are not established but the changes observed are consistent with the effects of adrenocortical hormones known to be liberated during stress. Vital capacity and venous pressure at rest and after exercise are normal, and so no possibility of significant cardiac or pulmonary insufficiency need be considered. The exertional dyspnea of emotion is based upon impairment of lactic acid metabolism and the fact that neurotic patients are discomforted more than normal subjects by visceral symptoms. These mechanisms, important in neurosis or emotional upset in normal subjects, are all the more so in congestive failure.

Emotional dyspnea, since it does not involve stasis in the lungs or the venous system, is not associated with orthopnea, a fact useful in differential diagnosis. Patients with neurocirculatory asthenia may do large amounts of hard labor under some circumstances and need not show the excessive prostration exhibited by patients with congestive failure who attempt exertion beyond their capacities; as a rule, however, emotional dyspnea causes enough disability to force the patient into some limitation of activity. Nevertheless there is no harm in the patient's exceeding what he believes to be his capacity for excerise. Misdiagnosing the condition as myocardial insufficiency may do harm to a nervous patient if marked revision of way of life is advised.

Some Metabolic Effects of Emotion

Metabolic disturbances found in emotional disorders are numerous and complex; many are not pertinent to the present discussion and only three will be considered.

An extensive literature, based on work in animals, has shown that discomfort or emotional stress stimulates the hypothalamic center that regulates the function of the hypophysis and results in liberation of antidiuretic hormone. This effect is shortlived in normal animals but excretion or inactivation of this hormone is slowed in the presence of liver damage, such as exists in congestive failure. That some edematous cardiac patients retain more water than salt is recognized, and this finding suggests the importance of antidiuretic hormonal effects as a mechanism of edema formation in heart disease. Patients with congestive failure regularly exhibit retardation of water diuresis as do patients with mental disturbances also.[29] Patients with mental disorders also show abnormally small responses to the injection of diuretic drugs.[29] The above discussion regarding one possible relation between emotion and exacerbation of edema in heart disease is largely theoretic and is designed only to call attention to the problem.

Patients with emotional disorders show many evidences of increased activity of pituitary-adrenocortical mechanisms. It has been shown also that distressing thoughts are followed by physiologic evidence in normal subjects, of increased formation of adrenocortical hormones. That these hormones favor salt retention is well known and accordingly this phenomenon must be taken into account in consideration of those patients in whom diuresis with the commonly successful measures is unsuccessful.

One action of the adrenocortical hormones liberated during stress is to impair carbohydrate metabolism so as to retard removal of lactate from the blood. This mechanism is basic in neurocirculatory asthenia, as discussed above, but also must be of importance, when present in congestive failure, in contributing to dyspnea, since the lactate metabolism is already markedly impaired in myocardial insufficiency.

Comment

Physiologic effects of emotion on the circulation in health and disease are many and varied. Their importance lies in the facts that

(1) they may exacerbate cardiovascular diseases; (2) their manifestations may resemble those of coronary sclerosis or myocardial insufficiency and so lead to erroneous diagnosis, and (3) their occurrence may call attention to the presence of emotional disorders not previously recognized.

No comment has been made relative to the effect of disease itself in causing emotional upset which in turn acts unfavorably upon the initial condition; this is true when the condition is organic heart disease or cardiovascular neurosis. An example is afforded by Sir Walter Scott who stated, "what a detestable feeling this fluttering of the heart is . . . I know it is nothing organic, and that it is entirely nervous but the sickening effects of it are dispiriting to a degree." This problem involves one of the most important aspects of the relation between patient and physician.

The problems raised by emotional disorders are probably not more numerous now than they were in the past, although they are probably different in character. Psychiatric and other medical writings of the past, from those of Burton down to those of the present, recurrently exclaim at the rapid spread of emotional disorders consequent to loosening of family ties, disintegration of morals, loss of influence of the Church and deterioration of economic security. It is startling to find that Erb, for instance, used these same explanations at the turn of the century, a period which today is nostalgically considered to have been one of stability and contentment. It is difficult to accept the pronouncements of today's Cassandras regarding trends in the incidence of emotional disorders. The importance of neurosis may seem particularly large today as a consequence of the fact that measures are developed in rapid succession for the exact diagnosis and specific treatment of many diseases; no such measures exist in the field of emotional disturbances and so, by comparison, they cause the physician more perplexity and dissatisfaction than any other group of disorders.

Except for the fact that the cardiovascular changes in startle reactions are similar in nature if not degree in various individuals, no consistency is encountered in the occurrence or character of cardiovascular phenomena which may appear in relation to environmental factors which influence the psyche. The emotional significance of the environmental factor to the individual patient determines the occurrence and in a measure the severity of the response to it. On the other hand, except in a small minority of instances where the nature of the cardiovascular response to emotional stress is evidently determined by neurotic indentifications or by conditioning in the past, there is no indication as to the mechanisms which result in the appearance of each of the various types of cardiovascular change.

In spite of the lack of a body of definitive data explaining the mechanisms underlying the occurrence of emotional reactions, the reasons for their variations in degree and nature, and the manner in which they cause bodily changes, there is no lack of positive statements bearing on all of these matters in the current literature. Much of the current writing on mechanisms whereby emotional situations cause cardiovascular symptoms consists in validation by anecdote, and is no more conclusive in establishing etiology than the writings of half a century ago that regularly ascribed heart attacks to the eating of spoiled or exotic foods. Attempts to prove that specific diseases are associated with or the consequence of specific types of personality arouse skepticism because of their lack of control studies, the limited amount of data presented, or evidence in some cases that the author is ignorant of the criteria used in recognition of the disease in question. Concepts which relate specific illnesses to specific types of emotional conflicts likewise are not convincing in that they appear to be based on superficial resemblances of one or a few of the many characteristics of the clinical syndrome to one or a few of the many characteristics of the conflict; it is not established, moreover, that conflicts are single, simple and invariable, or that they can become known or understood completely. Symbolic explanations currently encountered in the psychosomatic literature also invite skepticism. Acceptance of symbolic formulations regarding cardiac symptoms require acceptance of one of two hypotheses: (1) that the heart is a thinking organ, a concept established in the minds of the ancients but not seriously considered in recent times since Vireý stated more than a century ago that the heart originates thoughts and sends them to the brain via the vagi, or, (2) that specific changes in cardiovascular function in emotion always are willfully selected (consciously or unconsciously) by the patient, a concept that has no basis in substantial evidence. Similarly, attempts to explain symptoms as the result of vagotonic or sympathicotonic trends in patients on the basis of reactions of the circulation to epinephrine, atropine, pilocarpine and to various maneuvers involving autonomic reflexes, are not grounded in acceptable theory and are vitiated by inadequate observation and circular reasoning.

John Hunter wrote "There is not a natural action in the body, whether voluntary or involuntary, that may not be influenced by the peculiar state of the mind at the time." It may be taken for granted that the course of any illness can be influenced by emotional factors, and accordingly the physician must seek evidence of their presence in every case. The lack of adequate data for systematizing information regarding reactions of patients to emotional factors makes it essential for physicians to understand in general what these factors might be and to learn as much as possible about the life and personality of each patient in particular. Evaluation of the significance of emotional factors and their treatment will test his every art, for there is no skill that can be learned quickly and precisely in these matters. Although the barbiturates and other drugs are helpful at intervals, they are less so, and at times may be harmful, in the long run. Circulatory disorders consequent to severe neurosis cannot, as a rule, be alleviated to any great degree or for any length of time without psychiatric treatment. On the other hand, the milder emotional disturbances aroused in normal subjects by ordinary vicissitudes of everyday life, and the somewhat more serious ones precipitated by serious cardiac illness, can be handled satisfactorily, if recognized, by the artful physician.

ACKNOWLEDGMENT

This work is from the Laboratory of Clinical Physiology, McLean Hospital, Waverley, Mass., and the Department of Medicine, Harvard Medical School, Boston, Mass.

REFERENCES

[1] ZIMMERMAN, J. G.: A Treatise on Experience in Physic, vol. II. London, Sydenham Society, 1872.

[2] LESCHKE, E.: Die Ergebnisse und die Fehlerquellen der bisherigen Untersuchungen über die körperlichen Begleiterscheinungen seelischer Vorgange. Arch. f. d. ges. Psychol. 31: 27, 1914.

[3] GRAHAM, D. T., AND WOLFE, S.: Pathogenesis of urticaria. Experimental study of life situations, emotions and cutaneous vascular reactions. J. A. M. A. 143: 1396, 1950.

[4] ALTSCHULE, M. D., AND SULZBACH, W. M.: Effect of carbon dioxide on acrocyanosis in schizophrenia. Arch. Neurol. & Psychiat. 61: 44, 1949.

[5] MITTELMANN, B., AND WOLFF, H. G.: Affective states and skin temperature: Experimental study of subjects with "cold hands" and Raynaud's syndrome. Psychosom. Med. *1:* 271, 1939.

[6] THERON, P. A.: Peripheral vasomotor reactions as indices of basic emotional tension and lability. Psychosom. Med. *10:* 335, 1948.

[7] BLOCK, W.: Die Bedeutung des vegetativen Nervensystems beim Zustandekommen ortlicher Erfrierungen. Arch. f. klin. Chirurg. *204:* 64, 1942.

[8] OSBORNE, J. W., AND COWEN, J.: Psychiatric factors in peripheral vasoneuropathy after chilling. Lancet *2:* 204, 1945.

[9] NAIDE, M., SAYEN, A., AND COMROE, B. I.: Characteristic vascular pattern in patients with rheumatoid arthritis. Arch. Int. Med. *26:* 139, 1945.

[10] GOTTSCHALK, L. A.: A study of conditioned vasomotor responses in ten human subjects. Psychosom. Med. *8:* 16, 1946.

[11] GRANT, R. T., PEARSON, R. S. B., AND COMEAU, W. J.: Observation on urticaria provoked by emotion, by exercise and by warming the body. Clin. Sc. *2:* 253, 1936.

[12] BOAS, E. P., AND GOLDSCHMIDT, E. L.: The Heart Rate. Springfield, Charles C Thomas, 1932.

[13] GROLLMAN, A.: The effect of psychic disturbances on the cardiac output, pulse rate, blood pressure, and oxygen consumption of man. Am. J. Physiol. *89:* 366, 1929.

[14] STEAD, E. A., JR., WARREN, J. V., MERRILL, A. J., AND BRANNON, E. S.: The cardiac output in male subjects as measured by the technique of right atrial catheterization. Normal values with observations on the effect of anxiety and tilting. J. Clin. Investigation *24:* 326, 1945.

[15] HICKAM, J. B., CARGILL, W. H., AND GOLDEN, A.: Cardiovascular reactions to emotional stimuli. Effect on the cardiac output, arteriovenous oxygen difference, arterial pressure, and peripheral resistance. J. Clin. Investigation *27:* 290, 1948.

[16] WOLFF, G. A., AND WOLFF, H. G.: Studies on the nature of certain symptoms associated with cardiovascular disorders. Psychosom. Med. *8:* 293, 1946.

[17] STEVENSON, I. P., DUNCAN, C. H., AND WOLFF, H. G.: Circulatory dynamics before and after exercise in subjects with and without structural heart disease during anxiety and relaxation. J. Clin. Investigation *28:* 1535, 1949.

[18] MAKINSON, D. H.: Changes in the ballistocardiogram after exercise in normal and abnormal subjects. Circulation *2:* 186, 1950.

[19] DUNBAR, F.: Psychosomatic Diagnosis. New York, Paul B. Hoeber, Inc., 1943. P. 343.

[20] FREEDBERG, A. S., SPIEGL, E. D., AND RISEMAN, J. E. F.: Significance of effects of external heat and cold in patients with angina pectoris. Evidence for the existence of a reflex factor. Am. Heart J. *27:* 611, 1944.

[21] BLUMGART, H. L.: The question of "spasm" of the coronary arteries. Am. J. Med. *2:* 129, 1947.

²² WARREN, J. V., BRANNON, E. S., STEAD, E. A., JR., AND MERRILL, A. J.: The effect of venesection and the pooling of blood in the extremities on the atrial pressure and cardiac output in normal subjects with observations on acute circulatory collapse in three instances. J. Clin. Investigation 24: 337, 1945.

²³ BRIGDEN, W., HOWARTH, S., AND SHARPEY-SCHAFER, E. P.: Postural changes in the peripheral blood flow of normal subjects with observations on vaso-vagal fainting reactions as a result of tilting, the lordotic posture, pregnancy and spinal anesthesia. Clin. Sc. 9: 79, 1950.

²⁴ BULBRING, E., AND BURN, J. H.: Liberation of noradrenaline from the suprarenal gland. Brit. J. Pharmacol. 4: 202, 1949.

²⁵ WHITE, B. V., JR., AND GILDEA, E. F.: "Cold pressor test" in tension and anxiety. A cardiochronographic study. Arch. Neurol. & Psychiat. 38: 964, 1937.

²⁶ CHAPMAN, W. P., LIVINGSTON, R. B., AND LIVINGSTON, K. E.: Frontal lobotomy and electrical stimulation of orbital surface of frontal lobes. Effect on respiration and on blood pressure in man. Arch. Neurol. & Psychiat. 62: 701, 1949.

²⁷ JONES, M., AND MELLERSH, V.: A comparison of the exercise response in various groups of neurotic patients, and a method of rapid determination of oxygen in expired air, using a catharometer. Psychosom. Med. 8: 192, 1948.

²⁸ COHEN, M. E., WHITE, P. D., AND JOHNSON, R. E.: Neurocirculatory asthenia, anxiety neurosis or the effort syndrome. Arch. Int. Med. 81: 260, 1948.

²⁹ HOFF, H., AND POTZL, O.: Untersuchungen uber den Wasserhaushalt bei periodischen Psychosen. Ztschr. f. d. ges. Neurol. u. Psychiat. 124: 200, 1930.

Index

Acetyl strophanthidin, for paroxysmal tachycardia, 69
Acetylcholine, 121
Adams-Stokes syndrome, 76, 110
Adrenal gland
  and atherogenesis, 27–28
  cortical extract from, 24
Adrenocortical hormone, and emotion, 131
Adrenocorticotropic hormone, and atherogenesis, 27
Aging, and atherosclerosis, 10, 28
Alloxan diabetes, atherosclerosis in, 23
Aminophylline, 83
  for acute left ventricular failure, 79
Anastomosis, pulmonary-azygos, for mitral stenosis, 92–94
Anesthesia
  for cardiac patients undergoing surgery, 107, 112
  ventricular fibrillation during, 113–114
Angina pectoris
  vs. anxiety pain, 125
  lipoprotein level in, and atherosclerosis, 43
Anoxia, premature beats due to, during surgery, 113
Anticoagulant
  following pulmonary embolism, 83
  in quinidine therapy for paroxysmal auricular fibrillation, 71
Antidiuretic hormone, and emotion, 131
Anxiety
  and blood pressure, 127–128
  and cardiac output, 123–124
  cardiac pain due to, 125–126
Aorta, atherogenesis in, 21
Aortic valve, stenotic, 110
Appendage, atrial, Aschoff body in, 100
Arrest, cardiac, 76, 113–114
Arrhythmia
  and emotion, 122–123
  procaine amide for, 74–75
  during surgery, 112–114

See also Fibrillation; Flutter; Heart block; Tachycardia
Arteriole, constriction of, during emotion, 119
Arteriosclerosis, and hypertension, 25
  See also Atherogenesis; Atherosclerosis
Artery, transfusion into, 82
  See also Coronary artery
Aschoff body, in atrial appendage, 100
Aspiration, of pericardial space, for cardiac tamponade, 84
Asthenia, neurocirculatory, 129–130
  cardiac discomfort in, 125–126
Asystole, ventricular, 76, 110
Atabrine, for paroxysmal auricular fibrillation, 72
Atherogenesis
  and adrenal gland, 27–28
  and aging, 10, 28
  cholesterol concept of, 10–11
  cholesterol-induced, 25–26
  and cholesterol-phospholipid ratio, 20–21
  coronary, 21
  and gonads, 29
  and hypercholesteremia, 30–31
  and hypertension, 25–26
  and pituitary gland, 27–28
  and vascular damage, 26–27
  See also Atherosclerosis
Atherosclerosis, 5–65
  and aging, 10
  and aluminum hydroxide gel, 20
  aortic, 21
  and cholesterol, 9–32, 33–37
    in chick, 12–31
    cortisone in, 27–28
    dietary, 6–9, 14–18
    and organ lipidosis, 30
    and pancreas, 23–24
    in rabbit, 12
    in serum, 39–65
    species differences, 33–34
    thyroid hormone in, 22–23
    and undernutrition, 15–16
  choline for, 19, 23

137

Atherosclerosis—*Continued*
  combined theory of, 27
  and diabetes, 23
  and diet, 6–9, 11, 33–37
  and estrogen, 21
  experimental, 9–32
    in chick, 12–31
    dietary cholesterol in, 14–18
    history, 12
    in rabbit, 12
    and thyroid hormone, 22–23
  and fat, 6–9, 17–18
  focal character of, 54
  and heparin, 40
  human, 33–37
  and hypercholesteremia, 52, 63
  inositol for, 19
  and lipids, 7–8, 39–65
  and lipoprotein, 7–9
  and lipotropic factors, 19–20, 23
  and myocardial infarction, 53–54
  and obesity, 6, 16–17, 33, 37
  reversibility of, in chick, 14
  and S_f classes of molecules, 39–65
  species differences in, 29–30, 33–34
  spontaneous, in chick, 17
  stilbestrol-induced, 18, 22
    in chick, 13
Atrium, appendage of, 100
Atropine, 77, 83, 113
Auricle
  paroxysmal fibrillation, 70–72
  paroxysmal flutter, 72–73
  paroxysmal tachycardia, 67–70

Ballistocardiography, and emotion, 123–124
Beat, premature, during surgery, 113
Blanching, due to emotion, 121
Blood
  cholesterol in, and hypertension, 25
  lactate in, in neurocirculatory asthenia, 130
  lipids in, and atherosclerosis, 39–65
Blood pressure
  and anxiety, 127–128
  in shock due to myocardial infarction, 80
Blood transfusion, for shock due to myocardial infarction, 81–82
Blushing, due to emotion, 121
Body weight, and atherosclerosis, 6, 16–17, 33, 37
Bradycardia, and emotion, 121
Brain, vasoconstrictor impulses from, 128

Carbohydrate, 24
Cardiac output, and emotion, 123–125
Cardiac rate, and emotion, 121–122
Cardiac rhythm, and emotion, 122–123
  See also Arryhthmia
Carotid sinus, pressure on, for paroxysmal tachycardia, 68, 70
Cedilanid, for paroxysmal tachycardia, 69
Chick, atherosclerosis in
  cholesterol-induced, 12–31
  spontaneous, 17
  stilbestrol-induced, 13
Cholesteremia, minimal, 30–31
Cholesterol
  and adrenal cortex, 27
  and atherosclerosis, 9–32, 33–37
    organ lipidosis, 30
    pancreas, 23–24
    species differences, 33–34
    thyroid hormone, 22–23
    vascular damage, 26–27
  in blood, and hypertension, 25
  dietary
    and aging, 28
    and atherogenic lipoproteins, 8
    in atherosclerosis, 6–9
    in experimental atherosclerosis, 14–18
    and lipoprotein levels, 60
    and S_f classes of molecules in serum, 39–41
  ratio of, to phospholipid, 20–21
  in serum
    and atherosclerosis, 34–37, 39–65
    in coronary artery disease, 43–52
    in xanthoma tuberosum, 52–53
  and species differences in atherogenesis, 29–30
Choline, for atherosclerosis, 19, 23
Circulation, and emotion, 118–134
Cockerel, stilbestrol-induced atherosclerosis in, 13
Cold-pressor test, in normotension with anxiety, 128
Commissurotomy, 96–97
Coronary artery
  atherogenesis in, 21
  disease of, and lipoprotein levels, 43–52, 56–64
  occlusion of. *See* Infarction, myocardial
Cortex, adrenal, and atherosclerosis, 27–28
Cortisone, and atherogenesis, 27–28
Cyclopropane, 112, 113

Decompensation, cardiac, 111
Desoxycorticosterone acetate, hypertension due to, in arteriosclerosis, 25
Diabetes, and atherosclerosis, 23
Dicumarol, following pulmonary embolism, 83
Diet
  and atherosclerosis, 6–9, 11, 33–37
    cholesterol-induced, 14–18
    human, 33–37
  cholesterol in
    and lipoprotein level, 60
    and S_f classes of molecules, 39–41
  fat in
    and atherosclerosis, 6–9, 17–18
    and lipoprotein level, 60
  rice-fruit, and serum cholesterol, 35
Digitalis
  for acute left ventricular failure, 78
  for congestive heart failure, 77
  for flutter, 73
  in quinidine therapy for paroxysmal auricular fibrillation, 71
  for tachycardia, 69, 75–76
Digitalization, of surgical patient, 108–110
Digoxin
  for acute left ventricular failure, 78
  for congestive heart failure, 77
  for heart failure with flutter, 73
  for paroxysmal tachycardia, 69
Diuresis, and emotion, 131
Dyspnea
  emotional, 124, 130
  management of, prior to surgery, 109

Edema
  and emotion, 131
  pulmonary, 92–94
Electrocardiography
  during cyclopropane-ether anesthesia, 113
  preoperative, 107
  in procaine amide toxicity, 75
  in quinidine toxicity, 74
Embolism
  pulmonary, shock following, 82
  in surgery for mitral stenosis, 99
Emergency, cardiac
  Adams-Stokes syndrome, 76
  congestive heart failure, 76–77
  fibrillation, paroxysmal auricular, 70–72
  flutter, paroxysmal auricular, 72–73
  heart block, 76

tachycardia
  paroxysmal auricular, 67–70
  ventricular, 73–76
Emotion
  and cardiac discomfort, 125
  and cardiac output, 123–125
  and cardiac rate, 121–122
  and cardiac rhythm, 122–123
  and the circulation, 118–134
  electrocardiographic changes in, 123–125
  and hypertension, 127–129
  and metabolism, 131
  and neurocirculatory asthenia, 129–130
  and peripheral vascular system, 119–121
  and sudden death, 126
  and syncope, 126–127
Empyema, tamponade due to, 84
Ephedrine
  for Adams-Stokes syndrome, 76
  for shock due to myocardial infarction, 80
Epinephrine
  for Adams-Stokes syndrome, 76
  for cardiac arrest, 114
  during cyclopropane anesthesia, 112
  and duration of stress, 128
  and emotional tachycardia, 122
Estrogen, and atherosclerosis, 21
Ethylene, for cardiac patients undergoing surgery, 112
Exercise, in emotionally disturbed subjects, 129
Eye, pressure on, for paroxysmal tachycardia, 68

Failure, left ventricular, 77–79
  See also Heart failure
Fainting, 126–127
Fat
  dietary
    and atherogenic lipoproteins, 8
    and atherosclerosis, 6–9, 17–18
    and lipoprotein levels, 60
    and serum cholesterol, 35–36
  neutral, 24
  in atherogenesis, 17
Fear
  and cardiac discomfort, 125–126
  and cardiac output, 124
Fibrillation
  auricular
    acetyl strophanthidin for, 69
    management of, prior to surgery, 109

Fibrillation—*Continued*
  paroxysmal, 70–72
  after thyroidectomy, 115
  conversion, 73
  ventricular
    Adams-Stokes syndrome due to, 76
    during anesthesia, 113–114
    due to atropine and prostigmine, 113
Flotation pattern, ultracentrifugal, 44
Fluid, sodium-containing, in post-operative management of cardiac patients, 115
Flushing, due to emotion, 121
Flutter, auricular
  management of, prior to surgery, 109
  paroxysmal, 72–73

G substance, 37
Gel, aluminum hydroxide, and atherosclerosis, 20
Geriatrics, and atherosclerosis, 10, 28
Glycoside
  for flutter, 73
  for paroxysmal tachycardia, 69
  See also Digitalis; Digoxin
Gonad, and atherogenesis, 29

Heart
  arrest of, 76
    during anesthesia, 113–114
  outpute of, and emotion, 123–125
  rate of, and emotion, 121–122
  rhythm of, and emotion, 122–123
    See also Arrhythmia
  tamponade, 83–85
  work demand on, during surgery, 106
Heart block, 76
Heart failure
  congestive, 76–77, 110
    digitalis for ventricular tachycardia with, 76
    and surgery, 107–109, 110
  flutter associated with, 73
  due to paroxysmal auricular tachycardia, 68
Hemorrhage, in mitral stenosis, 92
Heparin
  and atherosclerosis, 40
  following pulmonary embolism, 83
Hives, 121
Hormone
  adrenocortical, and emotion, 131

adrenocorticotropic, and atherogenesis, 27
antidiuretic, and emotion, 131
thyroid, and experimental atherogenesis, 22–23
Hydroxide gel, and atherosclerosis, 20
Hypercholesteremia
  and aluminum hydroxide gel, 20
  and atherosclerosis, 52, 63
  dietary-induced, 16
  and lipotropic factors, 19
  minimal, and atherogenesis, 30–31
Hyperglycemia, in depancreatized chick, 24
Hyperlipemia, and lipotropic factors, 19
Hypertension
  and atherogenesis, 25–26
  and emotion, 127–129
  pulmonary, and Lutembacher's syndrome, 92
Hyperthyroidism, and cardiac decompensation, 111
Hypothalamus, and vasomotor changes during emotion, 120

Infarction, myocardial
  and atherosclerosis, 53–54
  and emotion, 126
  flutter in, 72
    heart failure due to, 77
  lipoprotein level in, 43–52, 56–62
  and lipoprotein levels, 56–62
  postoperative, 114–115
  and quinidine therapy for paroxysmal auricular fibrillation, 71
  shock in, 79–82
Infusion, intravenous, for cardiac tamponade, 84
Inositol, for atherosclerosis, 19
Insufficiency, myocardial, 109
Ipecac, syrup of, for supraventricular tachycardia, 70

Kidney, in hypertension, 128

Lactate, in blood, in neurocirculatory asthenia, 130
Lanatoside C
  for acute left ventricular failure, 78
  for heart failure, 73, 77
  for paroxysmal tachycardia, 69
Lecithin, in atherosclerosis, 23
Ligation, of femoral vein, in pulmonary embolism, 83
Lipid
  in blood, and atherosclerosis, 39–65

deposition of, and vascular damage, 26–27
endogenous, 18
exogenous, 18
and species differences in atherogenesis, 29–30
Lipidosis, and atherogenesis, 30
Lipoprotein, 7–9
level of
and coronary artery disease, 43–52, 56–64
and dietary cholesterol, 60
and dietary fat, 60
in serum, and atherosclerosis, 39–65
and species differences in atherogenesis, 29
in xanthoma tuberosum, 52
Lipotrophy, in atherosclerosis, 19–20, 23
Lung
edematous, in mitral stenosis, 92
embolism, shock following, 82
Lutenbacher's syndrome, and pulmonary hypertension, 92

Massage, cardiac, 114
Mecholyl chloride, for supraventricular tachycardia, 70
Metabolism
carbohydrate, pancreas in, 24
and emotion, 131
Mitral valve, stenotic, surgery for, 87–102
Morphine
for acute left ventricular failure, 77
for paroxysmal auricular fibrillation, 71
for paroxysmal auricular tachycardia, 68
for shock due to myocardial infarction, 81
Mortality, in surgery for mitral stenosis, 99
Myocardium, 109
See also Infarction, myocardial

Neosynephrine
and cardiac patients undergoing spinal anesthesia, 112
for shock due to myocardial infarction, 80–81
Neurosis
cardiac discomfort in, 125–126
cardiac output in, 124
electrocardiographic changes in, 123
emotional tachycardia in, 122

heart rate in, 122
vs. neurocirculatory asthenia, 129
Nitroglycerin, for acute left ventricular failure, 77
Nitrous oxide, for cardiac patients undergoing surgery, 112
Norepinephrine
and duration of stress, 128
and emotional tachycardia, 122
for shock due to myocardial infarction, 80

Obesity, and atherosclerosis, 6, 16–17, 33, 37
Occlusion, coronary. See Infarction, myocardial
Opiate, in paroxysmal auricular tachycardia, 68
Ouabain
for heart failure
congestive, 77
with flutter, 73
ventricular, 78
for paroxysmal tachycardia, 69
Output, cardiac, and emotion, 123–125
Overweight, and atherosclerosis, 6, 16–17, 33, 37
Oxygen therapy, for acute left ventricular failure, 77–78

Pain
anginal, 125–126
due to anxiety, 125
Pallor, due to emotion, 121
Pancreas, and experimental atherosclerosis, 23–24
Papaverine, 83
Paredrine, 76
for shock due to myocardial infarction, 80
Pericarditis, tamponade due to, 84
Phlebotomy, bloodless, for acute left ventricular failure, 79
Phospholipid, ratio of cholesterol to, and atherogenesis, 20–21
Pituitary gland, and atherogenesis, 27–28
Pituitrin, and cardiac patients undergoing spinal anesthesia, 112
Plasma, transfusion of, for shock due to myocardial infarction, 81–82
Position, for acute left ventricular failure, 77
Pressure. See Blood pressure
Procaine
for fibrillation, 72

Procaine—*Continued*
  for tachycardia
    supraventricular, 70
    ventricular, 74–75, 113
Pronestyl
  for fibrillation, 72
  for tachycardia
    supraventricular, 70
    ventricular, 113
Prostigmine and atropine, ventricular fibrillation due to, 113
Pulse, emotion-induced changes in, 119, 122

QRS complex, and emotion, 123
Quinidine
  for fibrillation, 71, 72
  for flutter, 73
  for tachycardia, 69–70, 73–74

Rabbit, cholesterol-induced atherosclerosis in, 12
Renin, and hypertension, 128
Rheumatic fever, mitral stenosis following, 100
Rhythm, cardiac, and emotion, 122–123

Salt, and hypertension, 129
  in arteriosclerosis, 25
Sedation
  in paroxysmal auricular fibrillation, 71
  in paroxysmal auricular tachycardia, 68
Semistarvation, and cholesterol-induced atherosclerosis, 15–16
Senescence, and atherosclerosis, 10
Septum, atrial, congenital defect of, 92
Serum, 8
  cholesterol in
    and atherosclerosis, 34–37, 39–65
    in coronary artery disease, 43–52
    and xanthoma tuberosum, 52–53
  lipoproteins in, and atherosclerosis, 39–65
Shock
  in myocardial infarction, 79–82
  following pulmonary embolism, 82–83
Shunt, extracardiac, for mitral stenosis, 92–94
Sinus arrhythemia, and emotion, 122
Sinus bradycardia
  during cyclopropane-ether anesthesia, 113
  and emotion, 121

Skin, cooling of, and anginal attacks, 126
Sodium, in fluids, in postoperative management of cardiac patients, 115
Sodium Pentothal, for cardiac patients undergoing surgery, 112
Spasm, vascular, during emotion, 119
Species difference, and atherosclerosis, 29–30, 33–34
Standstill, cardiac, 76, 113–114
Stenosis
  aortic, 110
  mitral, surgery for, 87–102
Stenotomy, 96–97
Steroid, adrenal, and atherogenesis, 27–28
Stilbestrol
  atherosclerosis due to, 18
  thyroid hormone for, 22
Stimulation, vagal, for paroxysmal tachycardia, 68, 70
Strophanthidin, acetyl, 69
Surgery
  management of cardiac patients, 106–117
  for mitral stenosis, 87–102
Syncope, 126–127
Syrup of ipecac, for supraventricular tachycardia, 70

T wave, and emotion, 123
Taychycardia
  auricular, paroxysmal, 67–70
  emotional, 122
  ventricular, 73–76
    Adams-Stokes syndrome due to, 76
    during anesthesia, 113
    during exercise in neurotic subject, 129
Tamponade, cardiac, 83–85
Thrombosis, coronary. *See* Infarction, myocardial
Thyroid hormone, and experimental atherogenesis, 22–23
Thyroidectomy, auricular fibrillation after, 115
Toxicity
  due to procaine amide, 75
  due to quinidine, 74
Transfusion, for shock due to myocardial infarction, 81–82

Undernutrition, and cholesterol-induced atherosclerosis, 15–16
Urticaria, 121

Vagus nerve, stimulation of, for paroxysmal tachycardia, 68, 70
Valve
  aortic, 110
  mitral, surgery for stenosis of, 87–102
Valvuloplasty, finger-fracture, 96–97
Valvulotomy, mitral, 87–91, 96–99
Vascular system
  damage to, and atherogenesis, 26–27
  peripheral, emotion-induced changes in, 119–121
Vasoconstriction, and emotion, 119–121
Vasodilatation, and emotion, 121
Vasodilator drug, for shock following pulmonary embolism, 82–83

Vasomotion, and emotion, 119–121
Vein
  bronchial, in mitral stenosis, 92
  femoral, ligation of, in pulmonary embolism, 83
Ventricle
  asystole, 76, 110
  left, failure of, 77–79
  tachycardia, 73–76, 113
Venule, constriction of during emotion, 119
Vomiting, for supraventricular tachycardia, 68, 70

Xanthoma tuberosum, 52–53